CAN FOOD BE MEDICINE AGAINST CANCER?

DR DAVID WILKINSON

The content of this book does not replace the advice and care of a health-care provider, and is not intended to provide specific advice for particular individual circumstances. It should not be relied on as the basis for any decision to take action or not take action on any matter which it covers. You should always seek the guidance of a qualified health professional for all health related matters. Any and all advice taken or applied from this book is the full responsibility of the reader.

Publisher:
Inspiring Publishers
P.O. Box 159 Calwell ACT Australia 2905
Email: publishaspg@gmail.com
http://www.inspiringpublishers.com

National Library of Australia Cataloguing-in-Publication entry.

Author: Wilkinson, David

Title: **Can food be medicine against cancer?:**
A healthy handbook that combines science,
medicine and not-so-common sense*/Dr David Wilkinson.*

ISBN: 9781925152234 (pbk)

Subjects: Cancer–Prevention.
Cancer–Diet therapy.
Cancer–Nutritional aspects.
Diet in disease.

Dewey Number: 616.994

Acknowledgement

Thank you most of all to my wife Helen who inspired me, both to start and finish the job! Thanks also to my colleague Dr Joanna Tait and my former assistant Marie-Lynn Castaing. They have all provided enthusiastic encouragement and feedback, ever since I embarked on this project some years ago.

A big cheer for the talent of illustrator, Bettina Guthridge, who wanted to contribute to the fight, and has done so in an insightful and entertaining way.

Ryan McDonald-Smith at Younique Creation was enthusiastic in designing the cover, and made some really excellent suggestions.

To my patients, thank you for allowing me the privilege of caring for you. I hope this provides you with the information, motivation and ultimately, the results you need.

Welcome to the reader. Purpose of the book. Who it is for.

Congratulations!

The fact that you are reading this paragraph means that you are interested in your health. You want some information. You are deciding what action you can take. Maybe you have had cancer or someone you know has had cancer or you just want to prevent it. In any case, I'm sure there will be something here for you in a format that you can access easily and apply immediately. There are a number of good books on this subject, but some are too cumbersome or too wordy, and not very user-friendly. Others are too superficial, or not based on evidence. Nutrition against cancer is an enormous subject in which it is all too easy to become lost. There are different opinions on certain matters which can entangle us and waste time. This book is not a comprehensive, all-inclusive reference book. Instead, it has been kept succinct, with a simple layout, so that you can start taking action today.

The intention is for this book to be motivational as well as informative, and I think the best way to do that is to provide the evidence behind the material presented. Would you change your lifestyle on a rumour? Or would you prefer the information to be substantiated? I know that when I came across some of these studies, I was quite excited to find that the research is convincing. Why didn't I know about this before? Whatever the answer to that may be, I don't want others to remain in the dark about how everyday food can maintain a barricade against cancer.

The best time to work against cancer is when the disease is microscopic. Most of the research available refers to this category.

It applies to prevention of cancer in people who have never had it. It also applies to preventing cancer recurrence, after the actual cancer lump has been removed or treated in some way. Cancers can return if there are any microscopic remnants. These are frequently too small to be detected on tests at first, but enlarge with time. Patients with more advanced disease should also use anti-cancer nutrition.

Some people are anxious about finding the perfect diet. However, adhering to a strict diet does not cure every malady, and what helps one person may not work for another. Becoming stressed can be counter-productive, doing more harm than good. Food is just the first and most obvious weapon we have, complementing all other treatments.

The key is to start somewhere and be motivated to keep on doing it. We are advised to have a balanced diet and do moderate exercise, but it is more than just that. Every meal can contain recognized chemical substances, with scientifically identified actions, that make a significant contribution against cancer.

How to use this book

Each reader will have a slightly different focus, so the book has been structured to enable easy navigation to the parts which match your purpose.

If you simply want advice for practical application, read Part One. You can even skim through to the end of each chapter, which will have a summary of key points. Perhaps you will browse the other chapters and read whatever catches your eye.

If you have been doing your own research, and want to see more evidence, the other sections will appeal to you as well. A number of key studies are described in Part One (practical), but many more are in Part Two (a bit more science).

If you are a medical doctor or health professional looking for nutritional advice to pass on to your patients, but you also want to see the underlying biology and molecular interactions, you will find the whole book useful.

Relevant underlying cancer concepts are explained in Chapter 18.

For further reading or enquiry, for updated information, and food suggestions etc, there is an appendix with resources.

Go to it!

CONTENTS

Applying the plan

PART TWO: A BIT MORE SCIENCE

Research notes: Biology, chemistry and studies

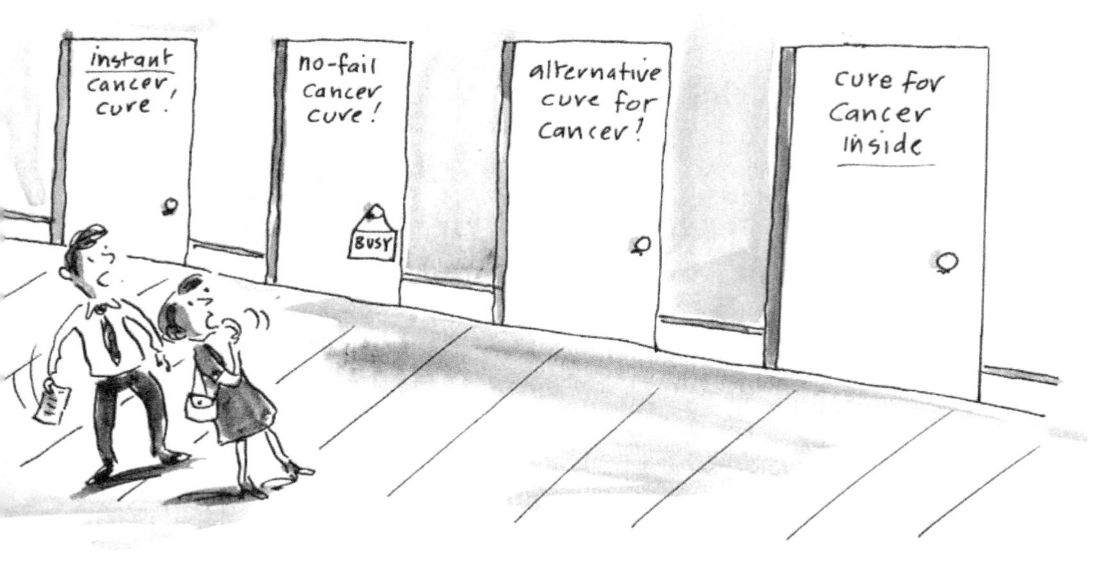

INTRODUCTION

The purpose of this book is to explore a core group of foods that work against cancer, and to provide enough evidence to convince you to adopt them as lifelong friends. These foods can then form a key part of an overall plan, together with other lifestyle components such as exercise and sunshine.

What Got Me Interested in this Subject?

For a long time, I was buried in my own little area which is the surgical side of cancer treatment. I naively assumed that someone else in the team was addressing issues like nutrition. And if no one was, surely that must mean that it didn't make any difference. Besides, anticancer nutrition was hardly mentioned in the text books, so I couldn't be missing anything important.

Like many of my colleagues, I have seen alternative remedies taken too far and fail tragically, when orthodox treatment would probably have saved or prolonged life. As a young surgeon I encountered a man with a bowel obstruction. Cancer had been diagnosed many months earlier at a treatable stage, but he declined surgery. Now he wanted help. In the operating room, when we opened his abdomen we found that the cancer was advanced, and the bowel itself was completely clogged with several kilograms of seeds which he had been eating to cure himself. On another occasion, a patient with breast cancer had surgery but declined any other treatment. Radiotherapy and an oestrogen-blocking drug were recommended, but she insisted that a plant-based treatment was more effective. The cancer returned as lumps on her chest and she died soon after. Unfortunately these and other stories like them deterred me from exploring nutrition as a weapon against cancer.

Then, a few things happened, and my perspective changed.

Firstly, a member of my own family was diagnosed with a chronic illness which essentially has no known cause and no known cure. I experienced the frustration of a patient (or relative) who tries to find answers outside conventional medicine. This usually means the internet, but also includes a huge array of books by all sorts of writers like patients, naturopaths, journalists and celebrities, as well as doctors. Even with my training and experience in medical literature and research, I was really challenged. If I was confused by it, I wondered how a non-medical person could make any sense of all the often untested and frequently conflicting information available. Were there any worthwhile gems hidden amongst the speculation and promises? I began to seriously empathize with patients who tried to do their own research with no scientific training.

I became aware of various diets and many confident but contradictory claims. I saw that cures were quite commercialized and everyone said that everyone else was wrong. I saw plenty of pure hype and wishful thinking, which my common sense and training taught me to disregard. Advice needs to be backed by evidence, or at least by honest and intelligent deduction, not based on the persuasiveness of smooth writing or the appeal of an anti-establishment philosophy.

As I said, a few notable things happened around the same time, or had my awareness just altered? I noticed that reputable sources were reporting that certain diets were resulting in less cancer recurrences. Some high-profile doctors diagnosed with cancer were speaking out for complementary treatments. My attention was drawn to some convincing books on the subject. For some time, cancer patients had been asking me what else they could do to help themselves. Now I wanted to give them a proper answer - one which I would listen to if I was the patient myself.

The Internet

The usual first port of call and in some ways the worst, is the internet. We affectionately refer to this as Doctor Google, and are all familiar with patients who come in armed with reems of downloaded information, wanting to know what it all means. The internet is flooded with ideas and claims, some genuine, some phoney, and many clearly commercially driven. Some sites provide useful information but may be too superficial. Other writers lack scientific training or thinking, and give advice based on philosophy or opinion, rather than evidence. Even so, statements on the internet have often prompted me to dig deeper and discover very useful information.

ASCO

At one of our oncology meetings, a colleague who had returned from the American Society of Clinical Oncology conference presented the findings of a study which indicated that a particular diet could reduce the rate of recurrence of breast cancer. This really startled me because we had rather ignored diet as potential therapy. Part of the reason for this is that medical specialists each have their own area of focus, and none of the team takes primary responsibility for lifestyle issues such as nutrition and exercise, which I now know are far more important than I had realized.

The China Study

As I was pondering food, a patient encouraged me to read "The China Study"[1]. In this book, Colin Campbell PhD makes some convincing observations regarding the link between cancer and what we eat. Also around this time, I found a number of studies demonstrating the importance of vitamin D in preventing cancers or cancer recurrence. Why hadn't I seen these things before? I was really learning something and it wasn't in the text books.

Doctors With Cancer in the News

Another firm knock on my door came when I began to see medical colleagues who were driven by first-hand experience to consider the role of food against cancer.

Dr Chris O'Brien was an Australian cancer surgeon at the forefront of his profession when he was diagnosed with a brain tumour. He underwent a number of operations as well as chemotherapy. Sadly, Chris has now died, but having experienced the limitations of conventional cancer treatment, he extended his therapy to include nutrition and meditation as well. He openly acknowledged that these had been under-utilized. Chris was enthusiastic about the development of comprehensive cancer centres that could offer complementary therapies alongside standard treatments[2]. Ironically, having treated other people's cancer with surgery for so many years, it was only after his own diagnosis that he began to explore other anticancer possibilities.

Dr Anna Donald, another Australian doctor, was an academic in the field of evidence-based medicine when she developed metastases (secondaries) from breast cancer. She had all the usual conventional treatments but, inspired by Ian Gawler, she placed emphasis on exploring meditation and spirituality, which she considered to be "a logical extension of scientific inquiry"[3]. (Ian Gawler was a young veterinary surgeon and athlete when he was diagnosed with an aggressive cancer which lead to the amputation of his leg. Despite receiving all the orthodox treatments, the cancer recurred as lumps in his chest. Against all expectations, he recovered through a number of means, including meditation and nutrition[4].) Anna lamented the fact that so little research goes into these approaches, stating that we do not know the efficacy of alternative treatments or how they work, because no one has studied them properly.

Dr. Mehmet Oz, a well known American TV doctor, became the subject of a recent Time Magazine article after he was diagnosed with a precancerous polyp in the large bowel[5]. He now promotes anticancer food on his website.

Dr. Richard Beliveau is a cancer researcher in Montreal. His passion for nutrition started when the parents of one of his very sick paediatric cancer patients begged him to use an intensive nutritional approach. To Dr. Beliveau's amazement, the treatment was effective, and he went on to make food a major focus of his research[6].

I decided that if these educated and respected doctors were taking this seriously, it warranted attention.

Is there Renewed Interest in Food and Cancer?

Have you ever seen something interesting that you have never noticed before, such as a certain kind of car on the road? Strangely, after that you seem to see them almost every day. Perhaps in the same way, I am now seeing integrated medicine organizations and anti-cancer diets all over the place. Even so, when I bring up the subject in conversation, people say they have heard little about it. The average person perceives that lifestyle factors are at best hopeful, but as you will see, the evidence for an actual measurable effect is mounting.

More Than The Big Three

"The Big Three" in cancer treatment has been used by some to refer to surgery, radiotherapy and chemotherapy. Patients keep asking me if there is anything else they can do, which is the question addressed by this book.

If there was another intervention which carried the potential of increasing the odds of surviving cancer, and which came at a relatively small personal and financial cost, shouldn't we be exploring it further and applying it?

As you will see from the studies presented, the statistical cancer survival benefits attributed to nutrition can be significant. Does that surprise you? Well it shouldn't, because our grandparents knew which lifestyles were healthy and which ones weren't. Today we think that the old-fashioned wisdom was not based on science, leading us to ignore it at our peril.

If we are prepared to undertake the ordeal of hospital treatments for cancer, why wouldn't we exert the necessary effort to adopt a lifestyle against cancer as well? The elements of such a lifestyle include diet, exercise and the mind. This book focuses on the first of these.

Food: How Does it Work?

You may ask how food could directly affect cancer. Don't we simply digest any food into its basic components, absorb them and reassemble them on the inside into the molecules we need? What exactly can specific foods do against cancer?

Consider the cause of cancer. I gave a presentation a few years ago and asked the audience which of the two was more important in the development of cancer: genes or the environment? Interestingly, a large number of them felt that genetics was the key factor. This is a very common misconception. Actually, genetic mutations only cause about 5-10% of breast cancers, and the figure is similar for other cancer types as well.

It's the Environment! (not Genetics)

Remember the nature versus nurture concept? What you start with in life (genetics) is nature and what acts upon that starting point is nurture (environment). If less than 10% of cancers are directly attributable to inherited genetic problems then the other 90% must be due to the environment. There is nothing else. During our lifetime, we are exposed to toxins such as cigarette smoke and mercury, and excessive hormones such as oestrogen, as well as carcinogenic substances in food additives, contaminants, pesticides and household chemicals. Imbalances in dietary fats, or deficiencies of particular nutrients can favour the growth of cancer.

We have focused on detrimental environmental exposure to toxins or carcinogens. We seem to have overlooked the fact that exposure to our environment includes what we take into our bodies as food, which can be either destructive or protective.

Cancer is a Multistep Process

There are a number of steps culminating in the presence of a life-threatening cancer. It starts with a normal cell which develops a mutation (i.e. a new mutation, as opposed to one we might have been born with). This leads to uncontrolled division and proliferation of the cell into a small cluster of abnormal cells. Further growth of these cells is promoted until it reaches the point where it requires its own blood supply. At this point new blood vessels form in order to feed the growing tumour. The next step is that some of the mutant cells develop the ability to penetrate the walls of blood vessels or lymph channels in order to enter the circulation. Not all cells that reach the blood stream lead to secondary cancers because, to grow into a new tumour, the free cancer cells need to lodge in tissues that provide the right environment for that metastatic cell.

Each step in the process is an opportunity to block the cancer.

Food as Preventative and Complementary Medicine

Food as medicine against cancer has a number of advantages.

Food contains a multitude of substances that can act against the different steps in cancer development, by a variety of methods. Some block environmental toxins from initiating malignant transformation of cells. Other plant chemicals inhibit the growth of new blood vessels into a tumour (angiogenesis). Still others promote the death of abnormal cells by programmed cell suicide (apoptosis). Specific food components stimulate the immune system, which helps to destroy malignant cells. Hence, we see that optimal nutrition strengthens the body's own natural resistance, as well as acting directly on cancer cells.

Food compounds act synergistically. This means that they act together to produce an effect that is even greater than just adding up the effect of each one on its own. You might expect two substances to provide double the impact, but with synergy the impact may be multiplied several times.

Another advantage of food is that you will be eating it for the rest of your life, compared to medical treatments, which have a limited duration. Every meal can be a cancer-fighting event.

Disclaimer and Warning

I do not claim to have read every significant piece of work on this subject or to have performed systematic literature reviews. That is not feasible for such an enormous field of research. I am happy to acknowledge that while we do see some negative or neutral studies, I have focused on those which demonstrate the positive results of nutrients against cancer. This approach is based on what I would consider to be adequate proof of mechanism, proof of concept and convincing statistical associations, as seen in laboratory work and epidemiological observations.

This book is not promoting food as a stand-alone cure for cancer, but as one of several pillars of resistance. There is no special diet that works for everyone, even though some people may have been cured of cancer while they were on a certain diet. Everyone is different with individual genetics and internal physiology, and cancers also vary considerably. Human beings are complex, with a number of intangible factors playing a part, including genetics, culture, personality, and stresses in life. Nutrition experts will disagree on some issues, and much is yet to be discovered or clarified. Reliable sources have been used for this book, and references are provided. Where significant uncertainty exists or opinion is given, it is expressed as such.

There is a wealth of information on anticancer food, but the other side of the coin is that it is impossible to keep up. This is not my primary field of work, and my aim has been to bring together what is becoming known, in an accessible practical form. If you are aware of updated information, please contact me for revision of future editions.

Always seek professional medical advice for your own specific circumstances. Diet does not replace conventional medical treatment. Don't try to cure your cancer with diet alone!

Part One: The Practical Part

The Top Ten

I have selected this group as the top ten based on the quantity of research and documented effectiveness against cancer. However, they are definitely not the only foods that have anticancer properties. They represent food components of different types with a variety of actions, and include food, drinks, spices, and supplements. They can be main meals, snacks or additives. I hope you will be inspired to utilize them.

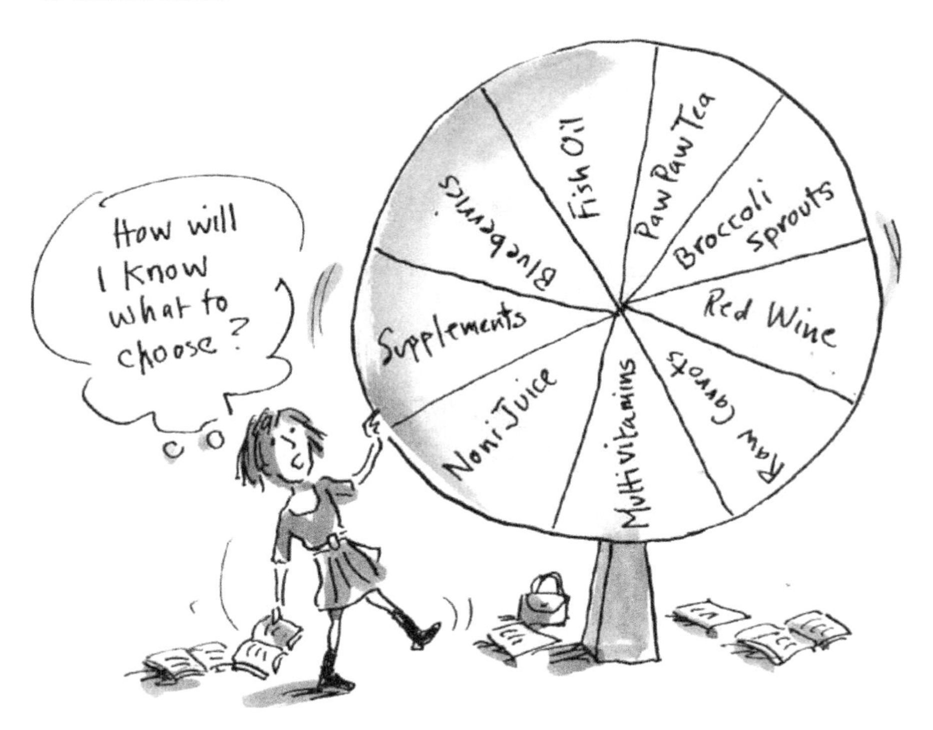

1. BROCCOLI AND THE CRUCIFERS

Broccoli is a great example of how much scientific information is becoming available in regard to phytonutrients (nutrients from plants) for cancer prevention. There may be more information about broccoli than any other anticancer food. Enormous amounts of similar data are now being accumulated on many other foods. By covering some details, I hope to give you confidence that an anticancer diet is scientific and not just wishful thinking. This will help you to stay motivated to make the necessary changes, particularly if you are at increased risk. Obviously you don't need to memorize chemical names or processes, but I think you will find the

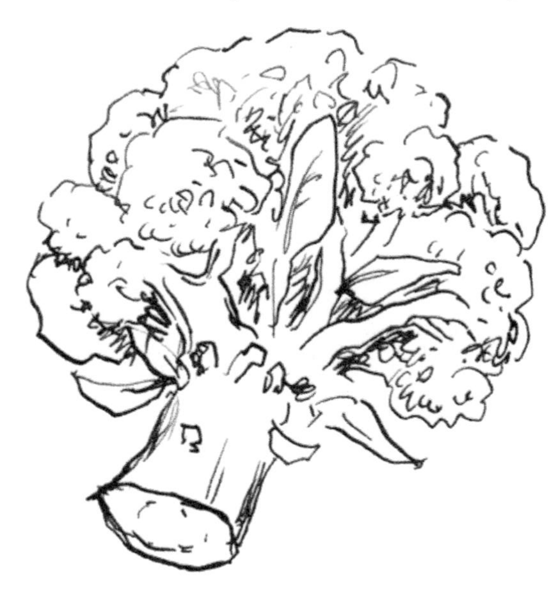

information interesting and persuasive. Common cancer concepts and biology mentioned here and in other chapters are explained in more detail in Chapter 18. Please just skip to the recommendations if the other details are not your cup of tea (there's a chapter on tea later).

Broccoli is in the family of crucifers or brassicas. Others in the family are listed in the table below:

Arugula (Rocket)	Daikon	Rape
Bok choy	Garden cress	Rapini
Broccoli	Horseradish	Rutabaga
Brussels sprouts	Kale	Tatsoi
Cabbage	Kohlrabi	Turnip
Cauliflower	Mustard	Wasabi
Collard greens	Radish	Watercress

As early as 1992, broccoli was discovered to contain specific nutrients that work against cancer[1]. In over 20 years there have been scores of studies regarding the effects of broccoli on cultured human cancer cell lines and cancers growing in animals, as well as various human studies. These look at the chemistry of the active components, as well as the measured effects of broccoli consumption on the rates of new cancers and recurrence of previously treated cancers. These studies are not always perfect in design, but are growing into

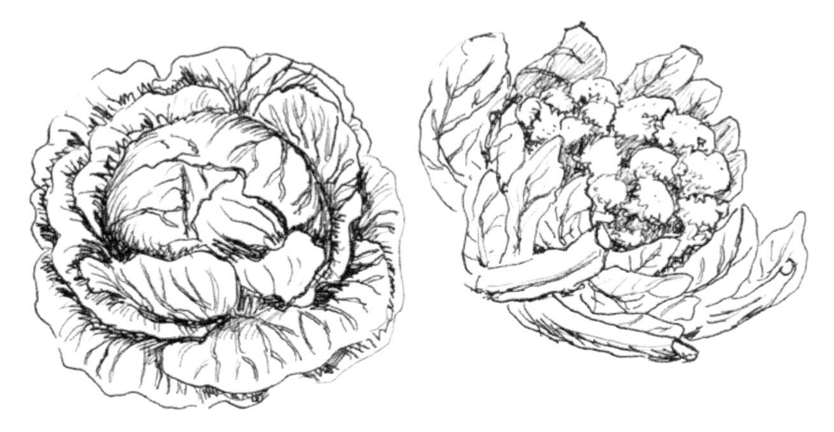

an overwhelming abundance of evidence which clearly adds up to something significant.

Studies on Broccoli and How it Works

For fascinating phytonutrients in broccoli, see Chapter 20 which also contains selected studies to provoke your interest and show you that there is plenty of scientific data.

The short version is that crucifers stop cancer cells from dividing, invading tissues, or gaining new blood vessels (angiogenesis, see below). They enhance expression of good genes, block oestrogen, and aid apoptosis (see below). The important nutrients are **indole-3-carbinol (I3C)**, and **sulforaphane (SF)** which requires the enzyme myrosinase for activation. The myrosinase is also contained within the broccoli itself (and in other crucifers) - how convenient!

BOX : DEFINITIONS - ANGIOGENESIS AND APOPTOSIS *(more detail in Chapter 18)*

Angiogenesis

"Angio" refers to blood vessels, and "genesis" means beginning or origin. "Angiogenesis" is the induction of new blood vessel growth which occurs in healthy tissue for normal growth, development and repair, but also in cancers. A cancer cannot grow beyond a tiny size without new blood vessels to feed it. Many plant-derived nutrients block angiogenesis in cancers without affecting normal tissue.

Apoptosis

This is programmed cell death. Cells which are abnormal, sick, damaged or no longer needed, have to be removed (especially cancer cells!). Our bodies have a built-in mechanism for this, called "apoptosis". Usual pronounciation is with the second "p" being silent.

These two terms appear repeatedly throughout the book. If they are new to you, just remember that, in the context of fighting cancer, angiogenesis is unwanted, and apoptosis is desirable.

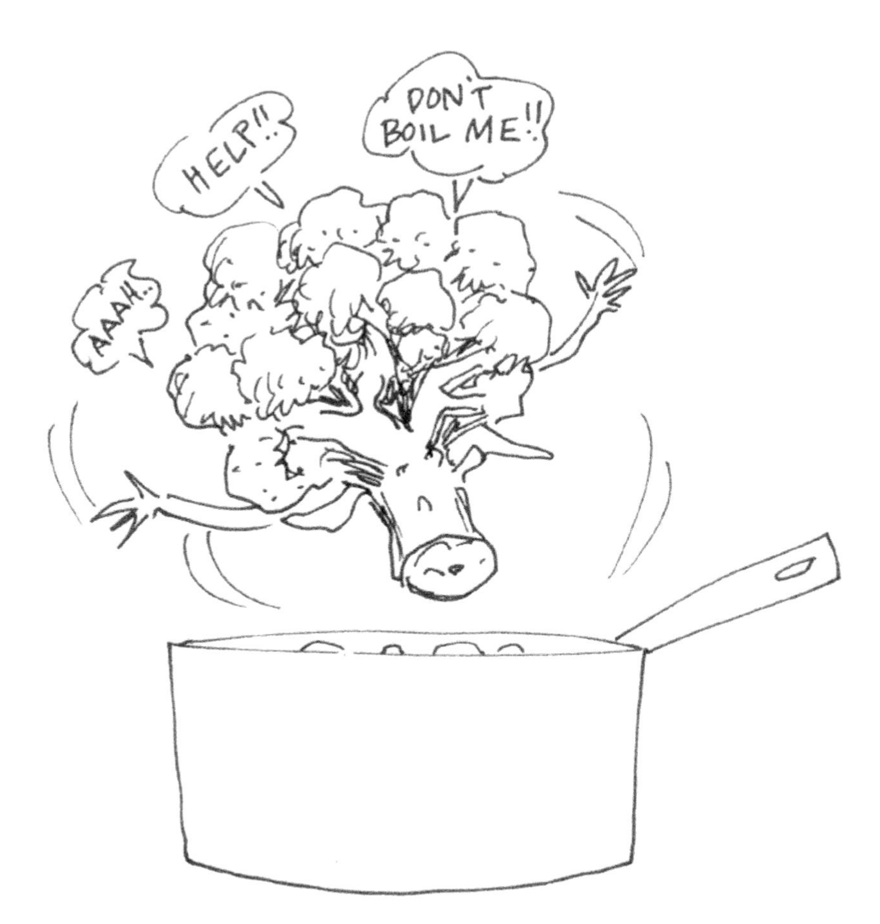

Preparation and Absorption

Cooking destroys the critical myrosinase enzyme[2]. Therefore, broccoli should only be lightly steamed. Three to four minutes of steaming may be even better than raw, because it blocks a protein in raw broccoli that interferes with the sulphur on the SF. Steaming for up to 20 minutes does not lower the levels significantly. However, boiling for just 5 minutes reduces the activated nutrient by 30%, and 10 minutes loses 50%[3]. If you prefer to cook it more thoroughly, have some raw crucifers as well to provide the myrosinase e.g. mustard, wasabi, horseradish[4]. Stir-frying is okay but should be brief (less than 5 minutes).

The important nutrients are stable to freezing[5], but deteriorate after prolonged storage, especially if pre-shredded[3].

Broccoli sprouts provide at least 20 times as much SF as the mature plant[6]. In sprouts, SF is dominant (90%), whereas in the mature plant, the indole type dominates (70%)[7]. Indole is the nutrient that has specific anti-oestrogen effects. So for many cancers, sprouts are a great idea, but if you are concerned about hormone receptive cancers such as ER-positive breast cancer, mature broccoli is advisable as well.

The myrosinase is only released when the plant cell wall is crushed, so chew it well. In fact, any plant foods should be chewed well because the cell walls are made of cellulose which we cannot digest. None of the valuable nutrients will be released from within the cell for digestion unless the cell wall is broken down (by chewing).

Phytochemicals at effective levels are easily measured in the blood, urine and body organs after eating broccoli[8,9] (Footnote 1). Blood levels are seen very quickly and significant amounts are in breast tissue within one hour[10]. Thankfully, it is not a case of requiring megadoses to produce a result in the lab and then finding you could not possibly eat that much.

Dosage – How much do I need to eat?

Based on published results, to reduce prostate cancer risk, three or more servings per week is effective[12,13]. For other cancers, five servings or more per week may be required[14-16], although even one serving per week is worthwhile[17]. A serving means half a cup, 125g, or four florets.

If you can grow or obtain sprouts, much less needs to be eaten. One ounce (25g) of sprouts results in as much SF as 20 ounces (500g) of a mature plant.

Other crucifers contain different proportions of plant chemicals in varying concentrations. Broccoli seems to be the best. The others are certainly beneficial in much the same way but perhaps to a lesser degree or with some differences in how they work.

I have been raving about broccoli since I discovered all this information, and I am amazed at how many people say they don't like broccoli. Is it because they overcook it? Just steam it lightly and have it frequently on its own or with almost anything. Retrain your taste buds if necessary; persuade yourself that it is wonderful and reap the benefits.

Footnote

1. There is large individual variability in metabolism of the nutrients. However, the SF causes induction of enzymes so that after a few weeks, twice as much can be measured in the urine, indicating improved blood levels[11].

Warning

1. Crucifers have high levels of vitamin K, and therefore may interfere with the medication warfarin (Coumadin) which is a blood thinner. If you are on this medication, and want to increase crucifers in your diet, do so gradually and have blood tests closely monitored.
2. The risk of blocking thyroid function by eating crucifers is very low, and really only applies to those who are iodine deficient.

Key Points

- Broccoli is the most studied crucifer but other common valuable ones include cabbage, cauliflower, Brussels sprouts, and kale.
- Broccoli should be cooked briefly e.g. steam for five minutes.
- It should be chewed well (to release and activate nutrients).
- Sprouts contain higher levels of one key nutrient compared to the mature plant.
- Mature (ordinary) broccoli contains more of a nutrient against hormone-sensitive cancers (e.g. ER-positive breast cancer).
- 3 servings per week will reduce prostate cancer risk.
- 5 or more servings per week advised for prevention of other cancer types.
- Serving = ½ cup or 125g or 4 florets.

2. BERRIES

Berries that have been studied for their anticancer properties include raspberries (black and red), blackberries, blueberries, cranberries, strawberries, and elderberries.

The best recognized substance in berries is ellagic acid, but in fact, there are a number of other elements in berries which work against cancer including anthocyanins, pterostilbene, quercetin, carotenes, and selenium.

Mechanism of Action

Ellagic acid is a strong antioxidant (see p.118).

However, berries are more than just a source of antioxidants. The anticancer effects of berries are also due to nutrients which have additional mechanisms of action.

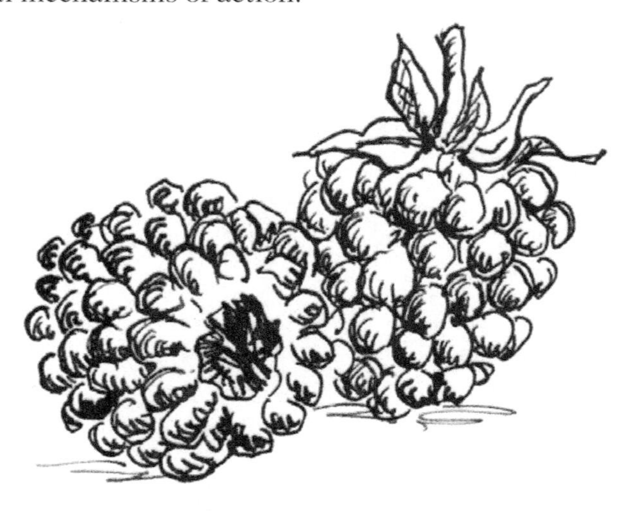

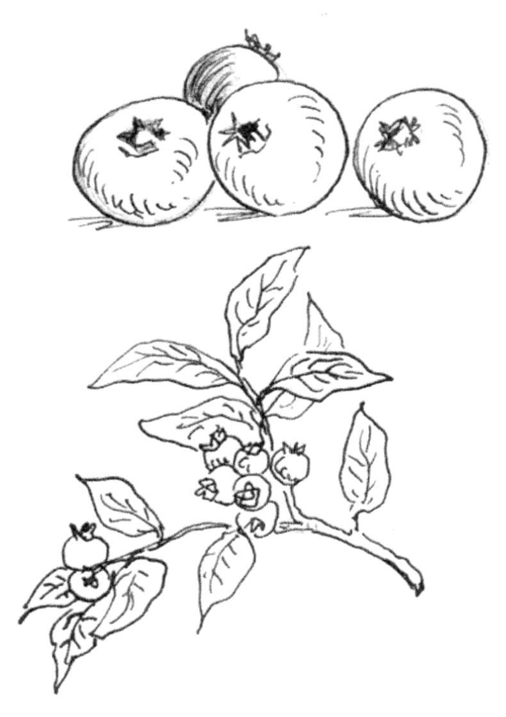

This has been shown by comparing the effectiveness of vitamin C (an antioxidant) with raspberries[1]. The raspberries were used at a concentration where they had less antioxidant power than the vitamin C, and still the raspberries were more effective than vitamin C against cancer cells. This demonstrates that there is more than just antioxidation going on. In other words, there are other components in raspberries that are blocking cancer (although the antioxidation helps too). Plants contain a variety of phytochemicals with very specific actions. If it was only the antioxidant power that mattered, you could just "dial up" a certain amount of antioxidants in your diet. On the contrary, we should eat a wide variety and good quantity of other fruit and vegetables to receive exposure to as many potentially helpful nutrients as possible.

Berries can also correct dysfunctional genes[2], block cell growth, induce apoptosis (programmed cell death of abnormal cells), inhibit angiogenesis, and suppress inflammation[3,4]. (These concepts are all explained in Chapter 18.)

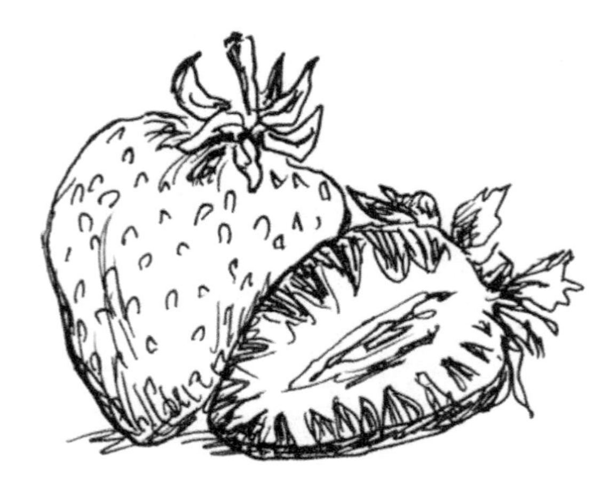

Research

The evidence that berry fruits have beneficial effects against several types of human cancers has been described in a review of the subject as "overwhelming"[5]. This is mainly in the form of laboratory evidence using animals or cancer cell cultures.

For example, in rats and hamsters, a berry-rich diet significantly reduced the incidence of colon cancers of the oral cavity, oesophagus and colon[6-8].

Cell studies in the laboratory have shown that berry extracts slowed the growth of cancers of the breast, colon, liver and cervix[9-12].

In humans, patients known to have precancerous lesions in the oesophagus were fed freeze-dried strawberries for 6 months. When re-tested at the end of the period, the majority were shown to have a decrease in the grade of their lesions (less aggressive and lower risk of malignant transformation)[13]. In a small study from 1985, consumption of strawberries appeared to reduce death from cancer[14]. There don't seem to be any more recent human studies with larger numbers which looked specifically at berries.

Which Berries are Best and How Much do I Need?

Interestingly, the less popular berries are actually more nutritious. For example, black raspberries are more seedy and less juicy than blackberries and are therefore less popular. However, the black raspberries contain more anthocyanins (as displayed by the darker skin) and probably more ellagic acid (being more seedy)[15], and will be more effective in blocking cancer. In general, much has been lost in the process of selective farming which favours appearance, texture and sweetness over nutrition.

Ellagic acid is found mainly in the pulp and seeds of the berry[16]. There is only a little in the juice. So don't just rely on drinking juice! Remember most commercial juice only stays clear and visually appealing because many phytochemicals (the key nutrients) have been removed, otherwise they oxidize and discolour the product as well as forming sediment.

Many of the other cancer preventers such as selenium, carotenes, quercetin and anthocyanins are also contained in the pulp and seeds.

Pterostilbene is a more recently identified player on this stage. It is found in blueberries, cranberries and certain grapes (e.g. muscadine and red grapes), although in relatively low concentrations. It is chemically related to resveratrol (Chapter 8). Pterostilbene is effective against breast, prostate, colon and lung cancer cells, synergizes with the breast cancer drug Tamoxifen[17], and may help against obesity-related breast cancer[18].

Elderberries may be useful against cancer because they contain immune stimulants and quercetin[19-21]. Only the blue, black or purple ones are recommended (not the red ones), and they must be cooked otherwise they cause nausea.

Unfortunately, a problem with berries is that it is difficult to achieve an adequate level of absorption into the bloodstream to be effective in all body organs[22]. The experiments mainly used freeze-dried powdered berries which have ten times the concentration of nutrients in fresh berries. Berry extract works against breast cancer cells in a laboratory dish, but it's no good if you can't absorb enough of it to reach a living breast. The reason why berries are mainly useful against cancers that arise from the lining of the digestive tract (oral, oesophagus, colon) is that the ellagic acid and anthocyanins come in direct contact with those tissues during passage along the gut. However, some ellagic acid is converted to urolithin which eventually reaches the urine where it can inhibit prostate cancer[23].

To provide an effective dose, it has been suggested that one cup of whole raspberries a day is enough[10,24]. Alternatively a supplement can be used but this should contain the whole berry or seed rather than a specific ellagic acid extract[3,25]. This dosage advice looks at berries in isolation, but it is important to reiterate that many phytochemicals from different plants work in synergy (see below), so they can still be effective in much smaller doses than expected. For example ellagic acid and quercetin act synergistically with each other and with resveratrol to induce apoptosis and cause cell cycle arrest[26,27].

BOX: DEFINITION – SYNERGY *(see p.105)*

Synergy means "acting together". It occurs when two or more components or substances work together to produce an ultimate effect which is greater than the sum of the individual effects. It's as if 1 + 1 = 3.

Summary

Berries work against cancer as antioxidants and by other important mechanisms. Large amounts would be needed if used alone, but sensible doses can be expected to be effective, particularly against cancers of the digestive tract, working synergistically in a diet rich in other plants.

Key Points

- Raspberries (black and red), blackberries, blueberries, cranberries, strawberries, and elderberries are all beneficial.
- They are effective against cancer as antioxidants but also by other important mechanisms.
- Berries with more seeds and darker colours contain the most nutrients.
- A whole cup of raspberries may be needed for an anticancer effect, but less would be required if the diet includes a wide variety of other plants.
- A similar dose can be achieved by taking a teaspoon of raspberry seed powder.
- The main benefit of berries is against cancers of the oral cavity, oesophagus and colon.

3. TURMERIC

What Is It?

Turmeric is a yellow/brown spice which is a common ingredient in curry, and contains the phytochemical curcumin. It is mostly available as a powder but is actually ground from the root of the Curcuma longa plant which is related to ginger and is prevalent in South Asia. You may see supplements labelled as Curcuma longa. Instead of buying the powder, you can buy the actual root and grate it yourself. Turmeric has been used for centuries in Ayurvedic (traditional Indian) medicine.

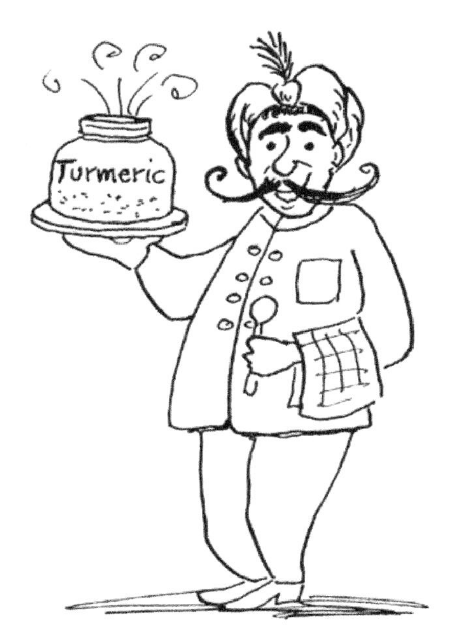

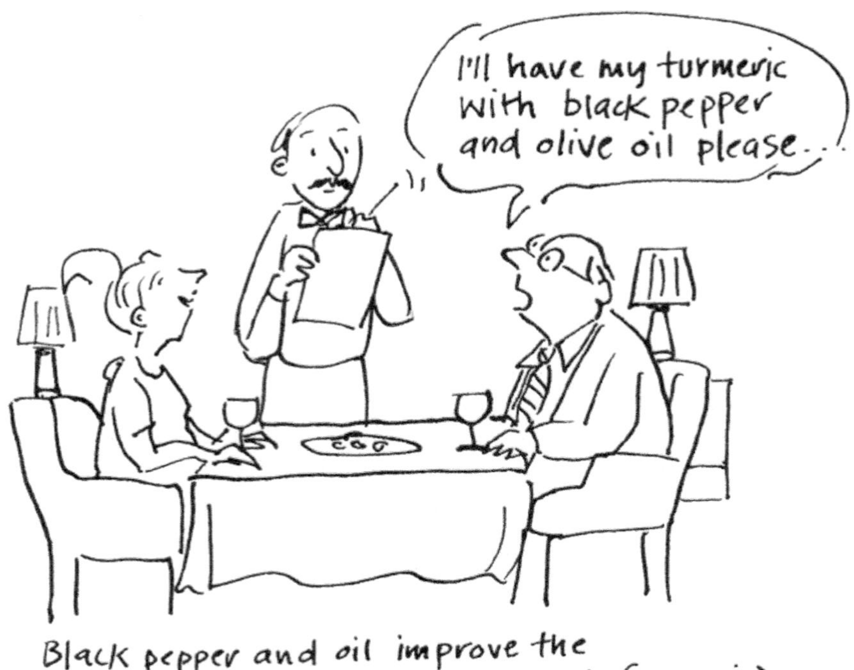

Studies

Cultures with a high turmeric diet have a lower risk of cancer of the breast, colon, prostate and lung. In India, where turmeric is a huge favourite, the overall cancer rate in 2008 was about 200 per million, compared to the USA where it is 600 per million[1], a three-fold difference although other factors such as lack of screening and under-reporting, are undoubtedly contributing.

There are hundreds of studies in animals and cancer cell lines, showing the effectiveness of curcumin against almost every type of cancer, with specific biochemistry being well-defined. Below are a couple of examples of human trials that have focused on bowel cancer.

1. Patients preparing for bowel cancer surgery were given 3600mg of curcumin per day for one week before the operation. When the tumour was removed, it was shown to contain significant levels of curcumin. However, levels of curcumin in liver

metastases (secondary cancers) were negligible. This suggests that the bowel received a good dose because of direct contact, whereas the amount entering the circulation was not enough to reach distant internal organs to any useful extent[2].

2. Patients with FAP (familial bowel polyps leading to colon cancer) were given both curcumin (480mg) and quercetin (20mg) per day for 6 months. When their colon was re-examined, the number and size of their polyps had decreased[3].

Curcumin has been favourably reviewed by some major research centres including the MD Anderson Cancer Centre[4], and results from more human trials are anticipated.

Mechanism of Action

Curcumin has been shown to block virtually every phase of cancer progression. This is detailed on p.127.

Effect on Chemotherapy

In most cases, curcumin may well increase the effectiveness of chemotherapy, and has promise against cancers which have become resistant to chemotherapy.

However, curcumin may reduce the effectiveness of certain types of chemotherapy. It would seem best to avoid curcumin while on particular drugs. See p.154 for details and other technical points.

Bioavailability

The main problem with curcumin is poor absorption. This is a disappointment since the anticancer effects in the laboratory are so well confirmed. However, there are ways to improve blood and tissue levels.

In particular, the combination of turmeric with pepper, oil and heat improves absorption and blood levels enormously. See below.

Synergism *(see p.105)*

The effects of curcumin are dose-dependent, meaning that the higher the levels, the greater the end effect. Because it is difficult to achieve high blood levels, we can take advantage of synergy to get the same result at lower levels. Do this by eating other foods which are known to amplify the effects of curcumin.

Curcumin is synergistic with resveratrol in grapes[5], EGCG in green tea[6], garcinol in mangosteen (against pancreatic cancer cells)[7], and probably others yet to be discovered. You probably wouldn't consume these together, but you could easily have them before or after a meal containing turmeric. Some people even tried adding a turmeric paste to green tea!

Side Effects

Doses of up to 8g per day have been demonstrated as well-tolerated and safe[8], but there are some areas of caution.

Possible interference with some types of chemotherapy has already been mentioned. Curcumin inhibits blood clotting and must be used with care in those taking blood-thinning medications such as warfarin or clopidogrel, and in patients preparing for surgery. It may aggravate gallstone problems, and can be implicated in iron deficiency anaemia because it binds iron.

Dosage and How to Take It

The fact that adequate blood levels are only briefly sustained, means that frequent doses would be required for a continuous effect. Some curcumin fanatics take it every half hour! However, it is probably not necessary to have a continuous peak level, and not possible anyway - while sleeping, for example. Those with active disease or metastases may want to have it very frequently, but those in remission or looking for prevention can simply aim for regular use to support other anticancer phytochemicals in the diet.

Remember that curcumin alone is probably quite ineffective because of poor absorption and rapid removal from the circulation. Therefore it needs to be combined as follows:

The simplest approach is to warm some oil (such as olive oil or coconut oil) and then add the turmeric and black pepper (contains piperine). A tablespoon of turmeric (about 7g of turmeric, which contains about 200mg of curcumin) is about right but if you are new to the taste, you may want to start with a smaller quantity. This paste can then be used with whatever other food is being eaten. It could be any curry, stew, soup, or simply mixed into rice or an omelette. It can be added to chick peas or lentils once they are cooked. The paste can even be used in a smoothie or just spread on toast.

In addition, the enhancer quercetin[3] can be taken with or 20 minutes before the turmeric, but the effectiveness of a supplement is not completely clear and I think it becomes over-complicated. Quercetin naturally occurs in onions which are easily incorporated into many meals anyway.

Several curcumin supplements are available, some plain, others with either oil or piperine added. Some have the curcumin encapsulated with a phospholipid to improve uptake across membranes. These could be considered if you have trouble incorporating turmeric into your diet, but bear in mind the pitfalls with supplements in general (see p.105).

Summary

The anticancer power of curcumin has been clearly documented in the laboratory with several quite amazing modes of action delineated in detail. The main hurdle is achieving adequate doses from diet alone. This can be helped by combining it with pepper and oil, as well as taking advantage of other synergistic foods.

Key Points

- Curcumin is the effective nutrient in the spice turmeric.
- It is active against many cancer types by several modes of action.
- Absorption is poor but can be improved dramatically by mixing with warm oil and black pepper.

4. GARLIC AND ITS FAMILY

This is the Allium group which includes garlic, onions, leeks, scallions, chives, and shallots. These add wonderful flavour to a huge range of food, and they fight cancer, too.

Chemistry

The chemistry of garlic is not only fascinating, but critical to how it is prepared for maximal effect.

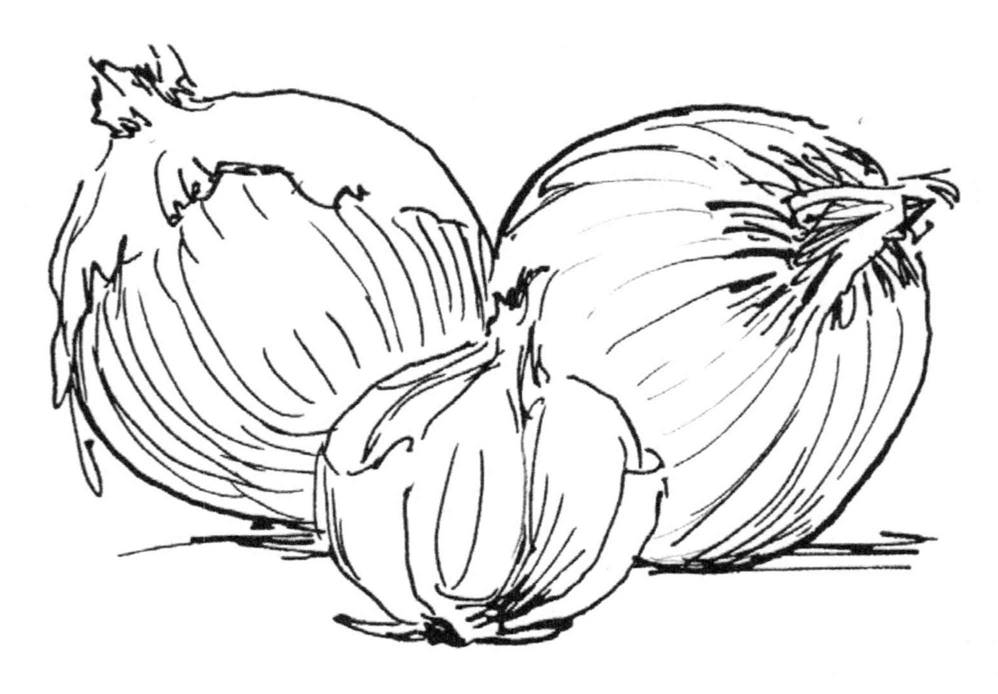

Allium vegetables contain:

1. Organosulfurs

The main organosulfur in garlic is alliin. It is converted to **di-allyl di-sulfide (DADS)**, which plays the key role.

The conversion requires an enzyme called allinase (or alliinase). This converts alliin to allicin which produces the characteristic garlic odour. Allicin is a potent cancer fighter but it is unstable and quite rapidly converts to DADS[1].

It is very important to know that the enzyme allinase is only released from the garlic when it is cut, crushed or peeled[1,2]. The more finely crushed, the more allinase is released, and the more DADS is ultimately produced. The chemical reactions are not instantaneous, and can only occur when the garlic is raw. Once it is cooked, the allinase enzyme is destroyed and nothing happens[3]. Most of the anti-cancer properties will be lost.

Therefore, wait 15 minutes after crushing before cooking (otherwise no DADS). Even after this interval, cooking will still reduce its

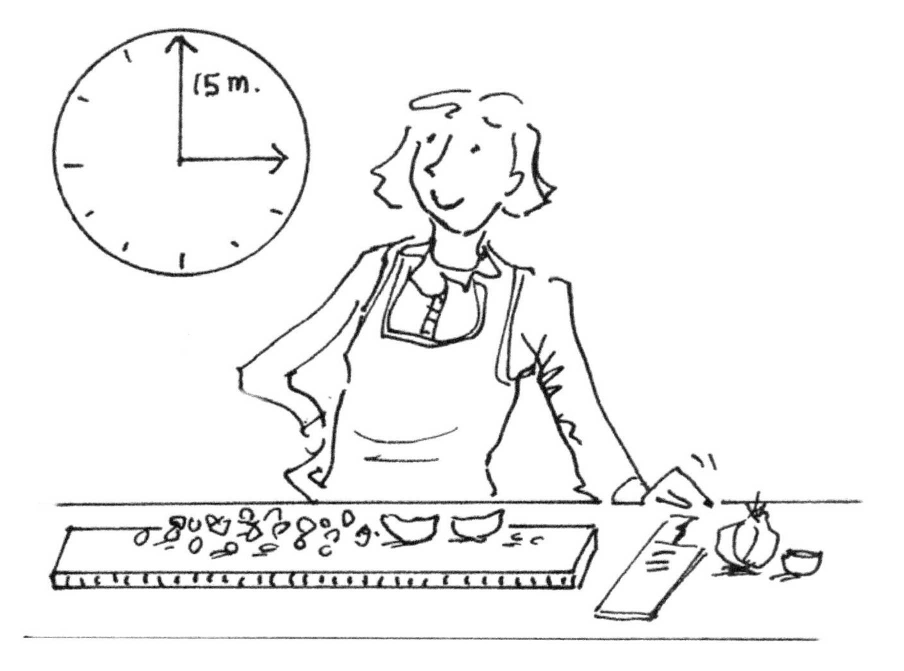

effectiveness compared to uncooked garlic, but only by about 30%. This is acceptable, given that most people prefer garlic cooked. The problem with eating raw cloves of garlic is that allinase does not survive stomach acid[4]. You would probably have to crush it manually, wait 15 minutes and then eat it raw to ensure maximal effect. Why not just cook it and use an extra clove to make up for the lost 30%?

2. Flavonoids

These include quercetin and anthocyanins, which we met in the chapter on berries. Anthocyanins provide the purple/red pigment not only in wine and berries, but also in red onions.

In garlic, the main focus is DADS, whereas in onions it seems to be the flavonoids, although garlic also has quercetin.

The various types of onions have been tested for levels of flavonoids with the following results[5]:

- red onions have the most, followed by yellow ones, and then white
- outer layers contain the most, with least in the centre
- shallots don't have as much flavonoid content but are higher in phenols (another phytochemical group), which gives them a stronger antioxidant ability than onions[6]

The strongest flavour indicates the highest chemical activity, whether it be garlic, onions, or shallots. This seems to be true of all vegetables with regard to health benefits. So don't go for sweet and mild.

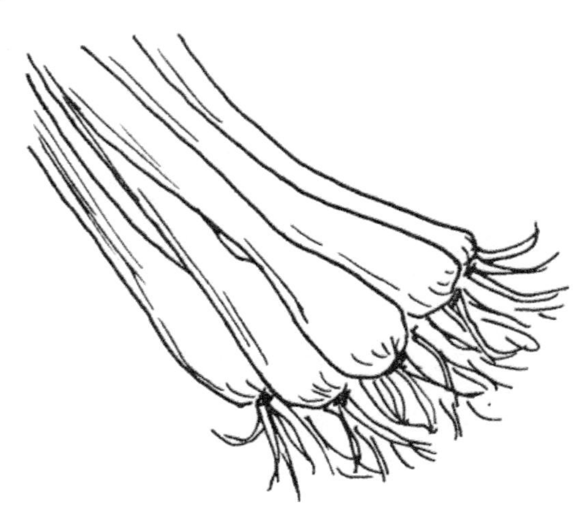

The "active ingredients" in onions are different to garlic, so they can be cooked straight away.

Mechanism of Action

Cells in a state of rapid division (such as cancer cells) are vulnerable to being destroyed. When cancer cells enter the stage of division to replicate themselves (which is what makes a cancerous mass grow), they become stressed. If DADS (from garlic) is present, it "freezes" cancer cells in the process of dividing (cell cycle arrest)[7]. Then they can be removed by apoptosis (cell suicide).

Quercetin[8] and anthocyanins[9], particularly in onions, have various roles such as blocking angiogenesis, inhibiting cell proliferation, promoting apoptosis, and also protecting normal cells against cancer-causing environmental toxins.

Garlic also has antibacterial properties[10]. This may explain the reduction in stomach cancer which can be related to the presence of the Helicobacter pylori bacteria.

Evidence

There are hundreds of papers that assess the role of the allium family against cancer. I have summarized selected studies in the technical section. They certainly show favourable effects in animal research. In human population studies, we see reductions in many cancer types amongst those who consume the most garlic and/or onions, with garlic being the main focus. The risk reduction ranged from 10% up to 80%, with the common cancers reduced by 20-30% or more, which is quite considerable. This is only for actual garlic in food as opposed to garlic supplements, which were shown to be unhelpful.

Preparation

When choosing garlic, avoid those with green shoots as they are old and will be less effective. The most pungent onions and garlic should be used. This applies to organic produce as well. If you have trouble preparing strong ones, get someone else to do it for you, or wear goggles!

Remember to wait 15 minutes after crushing garlic before it is cooked. Thereafter, only a small loss of activity results from cooking. Onions retain their effectiveness with cooking unless they are boiled[11].

If you eat garlic raw, the odour can be limited by having it with peanut butter, cilantro or parsley.

Garlic can be taken by juicing 3-4 cloves in a masticating (slow revolution) juicer. Onions can also be juiced. If it is too strong, a little honey or apple juice can be added.

Allium vegetables are better than supplements which often gave no cancer reduction in reported studies. The exception may be aged garlic extract (AGE), containing SAMC which inhibits division of colon cancer cells[12]. However, once we interfere with whole foods we don't know what other unrecognized and potentially synergistic elements may be lost.

How Much?

In the Italian Swiss study[13], half a cup of onions per day was considered a high dose and protective against many cancer types, but a more moderate amount was also beneficial. Remember, red onions are stronger and you will need less. Likewise with shallots.

The dose of garlic needed to produce an anticancer effect, based on some of the studies above, would be 2g/d, which is one smallish clove. Aim for this as the minimum to reduce cancer risk, although in one study even one clove a week was helpful[14]. Larger amounts seem to be better.

Side Effects

Be aware that garlic is a blood thinner and makes blood clot more slowly, so avoid it in preparation for surgery. Also, it interferes with Saquinovir which is a medication for HIV[15].

Key Points

- Alliin is a critical nutrient in garlic, effective against many cancer types.
- The garlic must be crushed or cut in order to activate the alliin.
- Wait 15 minutes after crushing before cooking, to allow full activation.
- The effective dose is one clove of garlic, or half a cup of onions, per day.

BOX: IMPERFECT RESEARCH – SOME CRITICS ARE HARD TO PLEASE *(see p.134)*

The fact that not all the research is consistent and that the studies show variation does not immediately call them into question. It merely reflects the fact that there is great variation in individuals, and within and between populations. Of course, reporting of exact dietary intake will be inaccurate, and a diet will often combine onions, garlic, olive oil, etc. Which ingredient carries the greatest effect? How much is due to synergy (working together)? Did the person even know what was in the meal? One negative paper[16] reviewed the subject and concluded that there was no proven anticancer benefit from garlic, but the authors did not consider any of the animal and laboratory studies and dismissed many population studies as using poor methods. Humans won't be locked up and fed a certain food for 10 years while we watch to see if they grow a cancer.

Variations in protective effects can be due to differences in type or quality of vegetables, the way they are prepared, individual sensitivity or genetics, different cancer subgroups, and so on.

The studies may not be perfect but they do demand our attention.

5. GREEN TEA

Introduction

The main anticancer plant chemicals in tea are called catechins, including **epigallocatechin-3-gallate**, abbreviated as **EGCG**. Most of the focus is on green tea rather than black tea, and on tea as a drink rather than catechin extracts or supplements.

Human studies have demonstrated the effectiveness of green tea against cancer, and the laboratory is uncovering how it works.

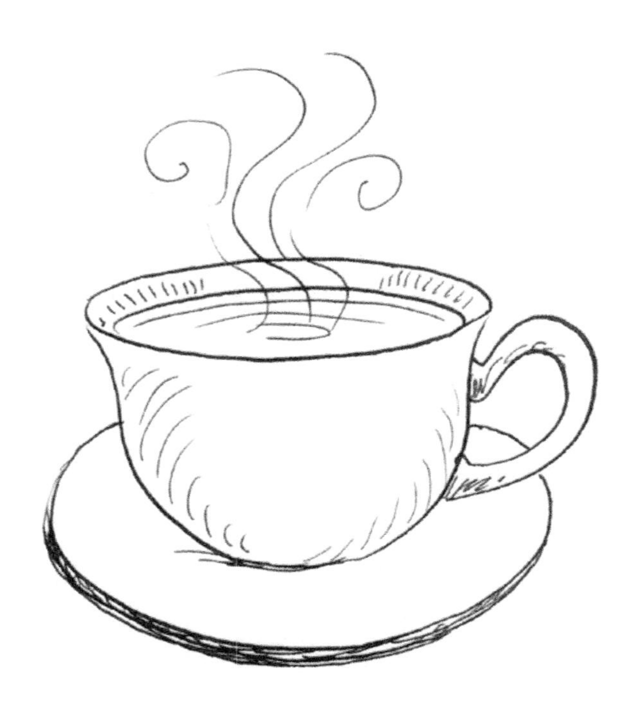

Human Studies

A Cochrane review of this subject was conducted[1]. It disregarded much of the evidence on the grounds of methodology, but even that rather negative review concluded that green tea decreases the risk of cancers of the prostate, lung, pancreas, colon and rectum.

Several studies are outlined on p.159. They are mainly from the orient (where they drink the most green tea). They include a mixture of study designs, covering a number of cancer types, looking at progression and recurrence as well as new cases. The results are remarkable, with risk reductions in the order of 20 to 50%.

Mechanism of Action

The effects of green tea on cancer at a cellular and molecular level have been determined from mountains of lab work on animals and cancer cell cultures.

The list of mechanisms (given in see p.161) is an absolute tour de force of anticancer weaponry.

Much of what is on the list relates to signalling pathways (see p.120). Growth signals have to reach the nucleus of the cancer cells by starting at the cell membrane and triggering a cascade of reactions which, like falling dominoes, eventually prompt the cell to divide or to develop more dangerous capabilities. Green tea blocks this chain of events at several points.

Green versus Black

Black tea here refers to black leaves (sometimes called red tea), not specifically to the style of having it without milk. The leaves blacken because they are allowed to oxidize (ferment) after being picked. The leaves contain an enzyme called polyphenol oxidase, which converts the flavonols into dark polyphenolic compounds (theaflavins), giving it the dark colour. Unfortunately, after this, only 15% of the cancer-fighting catechins remain[1]. Also, this type of tea is usually taken with milk. Milk may reduce effectiveness of tea catechins but this is debated[2,3].

Green tea leaves, in contrast, are subjected to heating which inactivates the oxidizing enzyme and so preserves the anticancer chemistry. In China, this is usually done by pan roasting while in Japan it is by steaming.

Decaffeinated and Bottled Tea

Does decaffeinated tea work? Decaffeination is commonly done by the ethyl acetate method which also removes 70% of the catechins[4]. Another method, using CO_2, retains most of the catechins, but how do you know which method was used? Tea chemistry is complex, so how can we be sure that a particular process is not interfering with other unidentified properties?

Don't expect much from bottled tea[5,6]. It will usually have a much reduced concentration of catechins (and is loaded with sugar).

Best Source

Be aware that tea quality and catechin concentration will vary according to soil, climate, fertilizers, etc. It has been generalized that Japanese tea is superior to Chinese, but that may be disputed. Usually the best quality comes as loose leaves rather than tea bags, and if not readily available from shops, can be ordered online.

Dose

A 120ml cup of green tea contains about 80mg of EGCG[7] (a lot less if it is decaff). This will vary widely according to type, quality, where grown, when picked, steeping time, water temperature, leaf size, etc. Using boiling water[8] and steeping (brewing) for over four minutes[9], will maximize catechin levels, although tea connoisseurs prefer (for flavour) to use water temperature below boiling and to steep for less than two minutes. The flavour may be better, but the health benefits are less. Subtle flavours are provided by amino acids and sugars, which are released early, whereas the healthy phenols (released with higher temperatures and longer steeping times) impart bitterness. In the studies that showed a benefit, method of preparation is not recorded. Whilst a shorter brewing time in cooler water for perfect flavour will be the aim of some drinkers, most will just allow the leaves to remain in the water for convenience. It is likely that a single stronger and perhaps more bitter cup (boiling water, longer brewing) may be as effective as several weaker ones.

In the studies available, the dose required for cancer prevention is as high as five cups per day (for oral, prostate, liver, endometrium) or as low as one cup per day (for ovarian cancer). Breast cancer risk reduction was achieved with over three cups per day. However, if you boost the EGCG levels per cup, by preparing it as above, fewer cups will be required.

Maximize Blood Levels

The bioavailability of EGCG is poor. Only about 10-20% reaches the blood[10]. This may be improved by three times if taken on an empty stomach[11] compared with having it with a meal. Absorption is further improved with sugar, vitamin C[10], lemon[12] or pepper. To be significant, this would require two teaspoons of sugar, 70mg of vitamin C, an equal volume of lemon juice (!), or 1.5 teaspoons of pepper. High sugar intake increases cancer risk, so try the other methods if you are game.

For maximal effect, a patient at high risk of a recurrence could consider having a strong/bitter cup and take the lemon, pepper or vitamin C as well, with a purely medicinal intent. However, for standard prevention, I wouldn't bother with this. The more complicated or arduous you make it, the less likely you are to actually do it. Just have green tea frequently for pleasure, on an empty stomach, first thing in the morning and between meals. Green tea is synergistic with curcumin[13], so if having a meal with curcumin (turmeric), the green tea should be had around the same time.

Catechins degrade in stored tea[14], so it is better to prepare and consume it fresh. Otherwise, vitamin C can be added to preserve the catechins for up to 8 hours[15].

Supplements

Supplements are usually ECGC alone, or as green tea extract which would include all the catechins, with EGCG making up about half. Some of these claim to have the equivalent of 50 cups of tea. The safety of such doses is unproven, and may be toxic to the liver. It would be sensible to use a dose equivalent to no more than ten cups of tea, perhaps up to 1500mg per day, or one capsule (300-500mg) three times per day.

Although EGCG is less bioavailable than the other green tea catechins, it is the most potent (Footnote 1). It does have synergy with the other catechins, meaning that it is more effective when they are present. This strengthens the argument for taking green tea as a drink rather than using supplements. If supplements are used, look for green tea extract rather than ECGC alone. As with other anticancer nutrients, the chemistry is so complex and incompletely understood, that we should adhere to the principle of consuming the whole food, with minimal processing, refining or other interference.

Adverse Effects

A cup of green tea contains 20-30mg of caffeine, compared to 50mg for black tea, and 100mg for coffee (but large variations for all). Decaffeination has two problems. Firstly, it removes most of the catechins. Secondly, it seems that caffeine itself contributes to the anticancer effect. In a rodent study, anticancer effects were not seen with decaffeinated green tea, but were restored when caffeine was added back in[16].

Tea inhibits absorption of non-heme iron when both are consumed at the same time[17], but not enough to affect the blood count. If this is a concern (e.g. in someone with iron deficiency anaemia), simply avoid having tea with meals.

Tea leaves concentrate aluminium from the soil, but the levels in tea are tiny (i.e. about 20mcg per litre, which means that you would need to drink 600 litres per day to breach the safe limit[18]).

Footnotes:

1. The other catechins such as EGC and ECG reach higher blood levels than EGCG. In rats, EGCG reaches its highest levels in the gut lining (oesophagus and colon), whereas EGC and ECG are better absorbed and hence detected in kidney, bladder, lung and prostate[19].

Key Points

- The main anticancer nutrient in green tea is EGCG.
- Green tea reduces risk by 20-50% for many cancer types.
- It works by blocking the signals which make cancer cells divide.
- Seek good quality loose-leaf green tea.
- Use boiling water and steep for 5 minutes (or just leave the leaves in the cup).
- EGCG is best absorbed on an empty stomach, but green tea can also be taken at meal times to achieve anticancer synergy with other food.
- Effective dose is 3 cups per day (more for some cancer types).

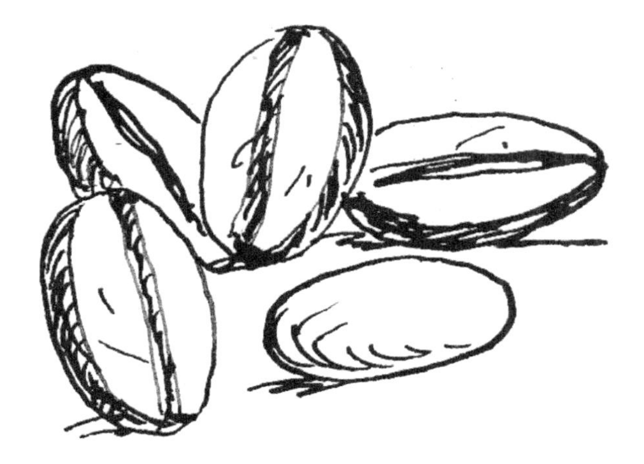

BOX: COFFEE

Coffee has previously been considered to increase the risk of some cancers. Many people seem to expect that because they enjoy coffee and even see it as an indulgence, it must surely be bad!

In fact, if anything, coffee protects against cancer. A number of mechanisms are possible, but it could be due to the antioxidant effect or to other specific effects of hundreds of phytochemicals found in coffee.

The exception was thought to be bladder cancer, but even this type was not increased until ten cups of coffee were consumed per day[20]. Furthermore, it has been suggested that the bladder cancer risk was due to the habit of coffee drinkers also smoking cigarettes. When the smokers and non-smokers are analysed separately, we see that coffee actually provides a protective effect. Smokers who drink coffee have a lower risk of bladder cancers than smokers who do not drink coffee[21].

One study showed that coffee is associated with a risk reduction for oestrogen-receptor negative breast cancer[22]. Another found that breast cancer patients who were on tamoxifen (an oestrogen blocker), had half the rate of cancer recurrence if they were coffee drinkers[23]. Perhaps everyone taking tamoxifen should drink two cups of coffee a day as well!

Endometrial cancers[24] and aggressive prostate cancers[25] also seem to be lower in coffee drinkers. Analysis of several studies concluded that in general, coffee reduces the risk of many cancer types[26].

The dose can be roughly quantified to some extent. Whilst for some cancer types at least five cups a day were needed, it seems that even two or three cups per day can be beneficial. Of course, there are problems which arise from too much coffee including anxiety, disturbed sleep and withdrawal effects. Less than six cups per day is suggested, meaning a sensible cup (8oz or 100mg of caffeine).

The data on decaffeinated coffee is lacking. Also, heavy coffee drinkers should bear in mind that sugar is a cancer risk and excessive dairy can be a concern, too. Beware of potential carcinogens in disposable foam cups, and of the chemicals in non-dairy whiteners.

6. FLAXSEEDS

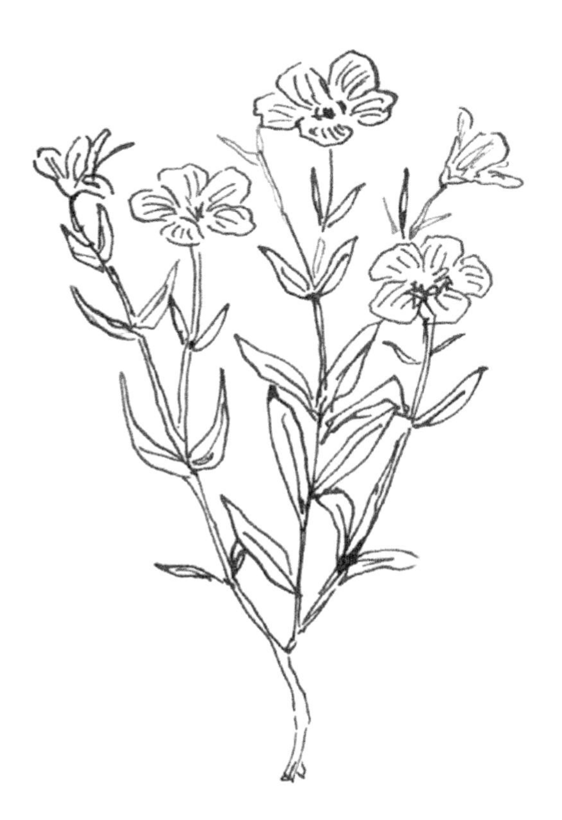

A single flaxseed is tiny but amazing in its contribution against cancer, containing both Omega 3 oils and lignans, each of which is independently effective. These two components tend to be studied separately, so the material is presented here in two parts.

OMEGA 3 OILS

Compared to other anticancer foods, omega 3 fatty acids have not attracted much attention and are better known for their role in heart health, particularly in the form of fish oil supplements. However, there is quite a lot of evidence that polyunsaturated fatty acids (PUFAs) are important in regard to cancer as well. The Budwig diet (Footnote 1) focuses on a combination of flaxseed oil and yoghurt or cottage cheese. The original research by Budwig is elusive, but there is evidence supporting Omega 3 oils against cancer.

Types of Oils: Omega 3 vs Omega 6

In regard to oil and fat, the experts continue to argue, and new information keeps appearing, so don't be surprised if you read differing opinions.

Here we are talking mainly about polyunsaturated fatty acids (PUFAs). They are grouped into Omega 3, Omega 6, and Omega 9 depending on their chemical structure. The "parent" Omega 3 (ALA) and "parent" Omega 6 (LA) cannot be made in our bodies and are termed EFAs (essential fatty acids). Fatty acids are needed for healthy cell membranes, and for the production of cell-to-cell messengers (cytokines) which have roles in inflammation, immunity, and cancer.

The modern western diet has drifted towards having a very high Omega 6 and low Omega 3 content. The Omega 6 oils prevail by a ratio of 20:1 or even more[1]. This is largely due to the move away from saturated animal fat towards polyunsaturated, which means vegetable oils and margarine (some margarines may also contain trans-fats – see Footnote 2). Probably for commercial reasons (i.e. cheaper crops to produce), these oils are predominantly Omega 6. In general terms, most Omega 6 oils are pro-inflammatory and undesirable in terms of cancer risk, whereas Omega 3 oils are protective. Of course, Omega 6 oils have important roles too, and should not be eliminated, but most of us do need to improve the ratio.

Omega 3 oils are from two broad sources:

1. fatty fish (e.g. salmon, sardines) or krill provide EPA (eicosapentaenoic acid) and DHA (docosahexaenoic acid).
2. vegetable sources esp. flaxseed (also called linseed) and walnuts provide ALA (alpha-linolenic acid) which can be converted after ingestion, into EPA and DHA

Almost all the other food oils are mainly Omega 6.

Natural oil sources contain a mixture of the oils in varying ratios, with most of them being dominated by Omega 6. The Omega 6: Omega 3 ratios are - canola 2:1, soybean 7:1, safflower oil 14:1, corn oil 50:1, and sunflower 70:1. Peanut oil has virtually no Omega 3. The canola ratio is better than the others, but its use is probably best minimized for other reasons (Footnote 3). It is the ratio in a person's total diet that matters, rather than in any individual meal.

Fish versus Flax

There is some debate over whether we should obtain Omega 3 from plants or fish. Either source is acceptable, and of course, both could be used. If choosing marine sources or supplements, make sure that they are not contaminated with toxins such as mercury.

Flaxseeds, as well as being the key vegetable source of Omega 3s, have the added anticancer effects of lignans and fibre. However, to counteract all the Omega 6s we are exposed too, an actual liquid oil supplement may be useful in addition to the seeds.

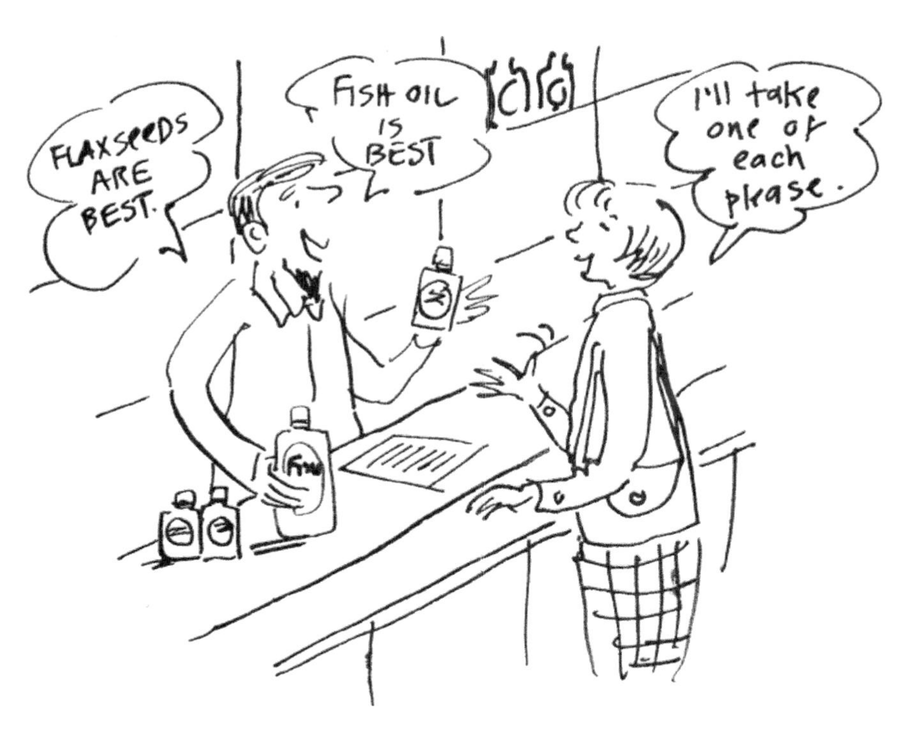

Animal Research

Chapter 25 (p.165) lists several rodent studies in which Omega 3 oils from fish, flax or walnuts were associated with less cancer, while animals fed Omega 6 from corn had more cancer.

Natural Fats versus Processed Omega 6 Oils

Although high fat diets in general increase cancer risk, some populations with a high intake of natural unprocessed fats have a lower cancer rate. For example, Eskimos and coastal Japanese people who traditionally consume a lot of fish and marine oils (high Omega 3 content), and Greeks and Spaniards who use large amounts of olive oil (mainly Omega 9) all have relatively low breast cancer rates[2].

So, some natural fats actually lower cancer risk, while standard vegetable oils (heavily processed and Omega 6 loaded), despite being promoted as healthy, may be just the opposite. Coconut oil is now seen as a healthy alternative to Omega 6 oils (Footnote 4).

Human Studies: Breast and Prostate Cancer

Several studies of Omega 3 oils have shown reductions in breast and prostate cancer risk.

Mechanism of Action

Amongst other mechanisms, Omega 3 oils suppress inflammation, block cancer cell migration, promote apoptosis of cancer cells, and synergize with the breast cancer drug Herceptin.

LIGNANS

We have covered flaxseeds as a source of Omega 3 fatty acids, but perhaps lesser known is the significant anticancer clout of their lignan content.

Lignans are present in many plants, but the concentration in flaxseeds is about a thousand times greater than anything else, except sesame seeds which have about one tenth as much[3].

In the bowel, lignans are converted by bacteria into enterolactone and enterodiol which are then absorbed and provide the cancer-fighting benefits.

Research

Animal studies have demonstrated the anticancer effects of lignans.

There is evidence in humans as well. Lignan intake, or blood levels of lignan products, are associated with reduced risk of cancers of the breast, prostate and bowel. In one study, survival amongst breast cancer patients was increased dramatically.

Mechanism of Action

Lignans block growth factors and angiogenesis, and promote apoptosis.

How to Apply this Information

Lower your Omega 6 intake

Minimize oils with high Omega 6 content including sunflower, safflower, soy, corn, and peanut oils.

Avoid commercial fried foods (Footnote 5), salad dressings, mayonnaise, and baked goods. Commercial preparations will usually contain Omega 6 oils.

Nuts provide many health benefits but most nut oils are mainly Omega 6. Balance this with a regular source of Omega 3s. The overall ratio in your diet is important.

Cook with walnut, olive, coconut, or avocado oils, or butter, rather than vegetable oils with high Omega 6 content. For high temperature frying, try avocado or rice bran oil.

What to do with the flaxseeds

Take two tablespoons of flaxseeds per day to provide an adequate dose of lignans and Omega 3 oil (Footnote 6). This can be boosted by a liquid flaxseed oil supplement (Footnote 7), or fish oil, particularly to offset any excess Omega 6 in your diet.

The seeds can't be digested whole, so they need to be ground. This is conveniently achieved in a coffee grinder. It is simple to have a small grinder just for the flaxseeds especially if you use it frequently, and then you don't have to worry about the flavour being contaminated with other grounds. The ground seeds should be eaten immediately, otherwise they go rancid and lose their powers (Footnote 8). For this reason, don't grind a large batch to use over a period of time, and don't buy pre-ground seeds. Even the unground seeds can become rancid. To prevent this they can be stored in an airtight container away from direct sunlight, usually in the fridge (as should liquid Omega 3 oils).

The ground seeds have a pleasant flavour, and can be easily added to a breakfast mix of any kind. It is worth making an effort to incorporate this into your daily routine.

Warning: Flaxseed oil (as oil) should probably be avoided in the last two trimesters of pregnancy as there may be a risk of preterm delivery, although flaxseeds themselves seem to be safe[4].

Footnotes:

1. The Budwig diet is a cancer remedy in which flaxseed oil is briskly stirred into yoghurt or quark. The liquid oil provides Omega 3s but lacks the lignans, so this can be improved by combining both the oil (Omega 3) and ground flaxseeds (Omega 3 plus lignans) in the same mixture.
2. Transfats are produced when vegetable oils are hydrogenated which makes them solid and easier to transport, as well as providing a certain flavour and crunchy texture favoured in many baked goods. They are an "edible non-food", providing no nutritional benefit, whilst increasing the risk of heart disease and possibly some cancers[5-7].
3. Canola, also called rapeseed, is virtually inedible without significant processing. It often comes from genetically modified crops, and dominates cooking oils due to commercial expedience.
4. Coconut oil was erroneously considered unhealthy because it is mainly saturated fat, but not all saturated fats are the same, just as not all PUFAs are the same. In coconuts, much of the fat is medium-chain triglycerides which are beneficial. They contain a significant amount of lauric acid which plays a role in the immune system. Coconut oil can be used in cooking, instead of high Omega 6 oils.
5. Apart from the Omega 6 problem, fried potatoes may contain acrylamide, a potential carcinogen that may increase the risk of some cancers, although the evidence is disputed[8].
6. The target for Omega 3 oils, from any combination of sources, is 4g per day (or more if you know you need to counter a high intake of Omega 6s). One quarter of a cup (four tablespoons) of flaxseeds gives 7g[9]. By comparison, one quarter cup of walnuts gives 2.3g (although walnuts actually have more Omega 6 than Omega 3). Fish provides 2g from four ounces of salmon. Olive oil is only 0.2g per ounce. Beef has only 0.12g per 100g (poor, despite the promotions by the industry).
7. Udo's oil is an alternative made up of a specific ratio of Omega 3,6, and 9 oils. If using marine supplements, 1200-2400mg of combined EPA/DHA is suggested.
8. Rancidification: Some oils, including flaxseed oil, become rancid (go off) quite easily when exposed to light or heat. The health benefits will be lost, and rancidification produces damaging free radicals. This

can be prevented by storing the oil in a dark container in the fridge. In contrast, extra-virgin olive oil keeps for a year, and saturated fats (including coconut oil) do not turn rancid.

Key Points

- Excessive Omega 6 oils are pro-inflammatory and linked to cancer.
- Reduce your Omega 6 intake by avoiding common vegetable oils and fried food.
- Omega 3 oils are associated with lower cancer rates.
- Omega 3 oils are found in salmon, sardines, flaxseeds and walnuts.
- Flaxseeds also contain lignans which have anticancer properties.
- Flaxseeds should be kept sealed in the fridge or freezer, and ground immediately prior to use.
- Two tablespoons of flaxseeds per day is recommended.

7. MUSHROOMS

Mushrooms have been considered to be of medicinal benefit for millennia, particularly in Asia. They contain many nutrients including vitamins, minerals, amino acids, fibre and compounds now known to be cancer preventive. One writer rather effusively declared that mushrooms are "miniature pharmaceutical factories producing hundreds of novel constituents with miraculous biological properties", and that they are "set to create a revolution in therapeutic strategies"[1]. They are immune-boosting, anti-nociceptive (painkillers), anti-diabetic, antiviral and antimicrobial. Their medicinal use has been termed "mycotherapy" ("myco" means fungus). There are thousands of types and there seems to be a degree of cancer specificity, meaning that certain mushrooms only work against certain cancers, and other mushrooms against

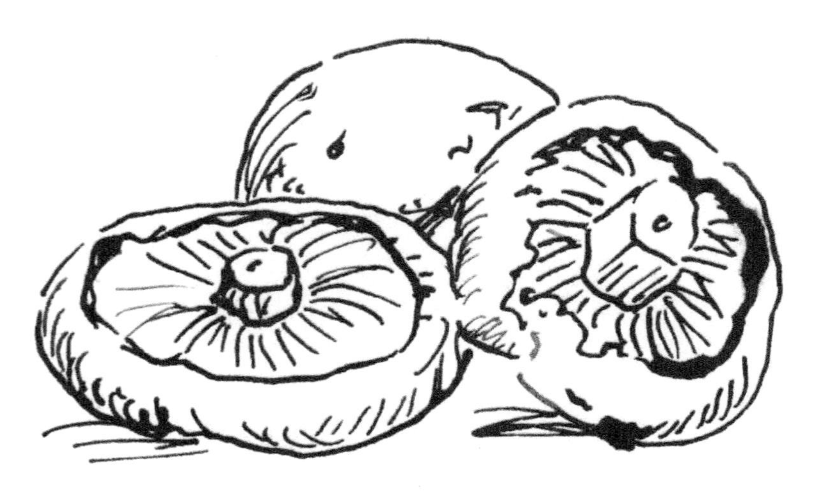

different cancers. Some require very high doses not achievable orally and have to be given by injection, while others are well absorbed and effective orally.

Why would mushrooms contain anticancer compounds? Mushrooms are saprophytic, which means that they live on dead and decaying matter. They produce growth inhibitors to combat competition from other parasitic organisms, in order to secure the nutrient-rich territory for themselves[2]. Those growth inhibitors can also inhibit cancer growth.

Here is a list of the commonly available and utilized varieties with the names of purified active compounds.

Scientific Genus	Common Name	Active compound or names of supplement
Pleurotus	Oyster	POPS-1, lectin
Agaricus blazei murill	ABM or ABE	
Agaricus bisporus	Button, table	
Agaricus compestris	Field mushroom	
Lentinula	Shiitake	lentinan (a beta-glucan), extract called SME or STM
Trametes* (or Coriolus)	Turkey tail, Yun zhi	krestin/PSP, PSK (polysaccharide peptide/K)
Grifola	Maitake	MDF (maitake D-fraction), also called PDF
Ganoderma*	Reishi, Lingzhi	RGM
Hericium	Lion's mane	
Cordyceps	Caterpillar fungus	cordlan, cordycepin
Flammulina	Enokitake, Winter	

*inedible (see below)

In the USA, the mushroom that is eaten the most is the Button mushroom (A. bisporus), which accounts for 90% of production[3]. Portobello and Crimini are other strains of A.bisporus. Shiitake, Oyster, Winter, and Maitake are popular in Asia.

The average Asian intake per capita is 11g per day compared with 5g in the USA[4]. I am surprised it is that high in the West, and I suspect that certain pockets consume a lot, while the majority consumes little.

Some medicinal mushrooms are actually inedible, including Ganoderma (Reishi) and Trametes, which are too coarse, hard or bitter, and can only be eaten when modified. Historically, they would have been used as tonics, tinctures, teas and powders. With regard to these types, it is fascinating to ponder how their medicinal powers were ever discovered, given that they are uncommon and only found in the forest.

Laboratory and Animal Evidence

As with other plants (although mushrooms are not strictly a plant), there is plenty of laboratory evidence for an anticancer effect.

In mice with sarcomas (aggressive connective tissue cancers) and liver cancers, Ganoderma extracts of different types caused a 90% reduction of growth[5]. Metastases (secondaries) and the ability to metastasize have been studied separately. Ganoderma suppresses migration and invasion by breast and prostate cancer cells[6]. PDF (from Maitake mushrooms) reduced liver metastases in mice by more than 90%[7].

Outside the lab, dogs diagnosed with haemangiosarcoma (aggressive cancer arising from blood vessels) were treated with oral supplements of PSP (extract from Coriolus or Turkey tail mushroom). In untreated dogs, the longest reported (maximum) survival was 86 days, but with PSP the median (middle of the group) survival was 199 days[8].

Epidemiological Observations

Farmers who grow (and presumably consume) Flammulina mushrooms in the Nagano prefecture of Japan were shown to have a significantly lower death rate from cancer compared to other regions (only 97 deaths vs 160 deaths, per 100,000 people)[9,10].

The Agaricus blazei mushroom is native to a small mountainous area near Sao Paulo in Brazil. The local population was noted to have a very low incidence of several diseases, including cancer[10].

Human Studies

As with many complementary cancer treatments, there are individual case reports with remarkable results, including patients with liver or lung secondaries which did not respond to chemotherapy, but disappeared after a course of Maitake mushrooms and its extract, MDF[11]. Patients with elevated PSA (a sign of prostate cancer) have seen it lowered by mushroom supplements[7].

Beyond this, there are a number of clinical trials and case control studies. Most of the published results are from Japan and focus on what is referred to as adjuvant immunotherapy, meaning that mushrooms or extracts (the immune part) are given alongside standard chemotherapy.

The mushroom extracts Lentinan and PSK both resulted in reduced recurrence rates for stomach and bowel cancer, including higher stage disease. In population cohort studies, those who ate the most mushrooms had less breast cancer.

Safety

There has been a perception that because mushrooms are fungi, they will increase the risk of "yeast" infections, but this is considered by most to be untrue. However, some fungi do cause diseases and some are carcinogenic. This may explain why there has been a degree of "mycophobia" in the UK, Ireland and North America, in contrast to much of Europe and the fungus-loving societies in Asia where they have been used for thousands of years.

See notes below on the dangers of raw and poisonous mushrooms.

Extracts used in clinical trials have shown virtually no adverse effects, including during pregnancy or lactation. In a Lentinan trial with 469 patients, only two patients discontinued due to side effects[10,12]. This is in contrast with other BMRs (biological response modifiers) used in cancer research, such as interleukin, interferon, and tumour necrosis factor, which can produce quite severe side effects.

Mechanism of Action – Immunity, Immunity!

A healthy immune system is not just for fighting infections but provides surveillance of the whole body and provides resistance to cancer. Cancer cells are abnormal and our immune system frequently recognises them as such, allowing destruction and removal.

Mushrooms contain beta-glucans, which activate the immune system.

In addition, mushrooms block oestrogen, inhibit invasion and metastasis, trigger apoptosis and may prevent recurrences caused by resistant stem cells. They enhance chemotherapy whilst lowering chemo side effects.

Dose and Type

The case control studies showed a reduced risk of cancer with an intake of at least 10 g/d, or a frequency of three times per week.

The best (and most studied) edible mushrooms seem to be Maitake, Shiitake, Oyster and Winter mushrooms which are edible and readily available. Agaricus blazei (not the same as other common Agarici) will not be easily obtainable except as a supplement. Trametes and Reishi are effective but inedible and have to be taken as supplements also.

Storage

It must be pointed out that the effects of Shiitake (and presumably the others) are retained if stored at four degrees, but mushrooms kept at 20 degrees for one week lose their effectiveness due to degradation by internal beta-glucanase enzymes[10].

Dried mushrooms are available and can be rehydrated by covering with boiling water and left to soak for half an hour. Squeeze out the remaining liquid but consider saving it for cooking. I could not find specific information on the preservation of beta-glucans in dried mushrooms. However, if they are dried soon after harvesting and kept cool, the beta-glucans should be preserved.

The concentration of beta-glucans depends on the stage of development of the fruiting body of the mushroom, being maximal during growth and diminished in final maturation[10].

Cooked versus Raw

While button mushrooms are often eaten raw in salads, it is advised that mushrooms should be cooked for two reasons[13]. Firstly, mushroom cell walls are indigestible. Cooking breaks down the cell walls, making the nutrients available for absorption.

Secondly, cooking destroys certain toxins in mushrooms, and reduces the risk of gastrointestinal irritation or allergic reactions. Agaritine is a substance present in all species of Agaricus (Button, Portobello, "field") mushrooms and it is only partly removed by cooking. Concerns have been raised about the possibility of agaritine being carcinogenic in mice. However, it is confirmed as non-toxic to humans. Of course certain toadstools remain poisonous even after cooking. Only mushrooms known to be safe should be eaten! Don't go picking and eating any old thing. Furthermore, mushrooms are frequently cultivated on horse manure and may be contaminated with bacteria that may not be completely removed with washing, but will be destroyed by cooking.

Supplements

The other way to take them is as a supplement. Perhaps consider doing this if you have an increased risk of cancer (e.g. strong family history) or a past history of cancer. This applies when you can't be sure of the quality or freshness of whole mushrooms or you just want to achieve a higher dose. Unlike other foods, in the case of mushrooms, extracts and supplements have been shown to be effective. Indeed several studies used them in combination with whole mushrooms or even alone.

Many commercial preparations are available[7,10]. A supplement containing a mixture of several different mushroom extracts has been recommended. For example, extracts from Agaricus blazei, Shiitake, Maitake, Tramete/Coriolus and Reishi. This has been termed "shotgun mycotherapy"[2], and makes sense because different mushrooms have specificity against particular cancer types. The terminology can be confusing, which is why I listed various interchangeable names earlier in this chapter.

Summary

Mushrooms provide us with an anticancer food working from a slightly different angle, one which focuses on boosting the immune system. In the kitchen they provide flavour, depth and variety, and should certainly be incorporated where possible. However, for those at high risk, also consider taking a supplement.

Key Points

- Mushrooms contain beta-glucans, which stimulate the immune system.
- The immune system plays an important role against cancer.
- Mushrooms are best if obtained fresh, stored cool, and eaten cooked.
- Those with a high cancer risk may consider using a supplement.

8. RESVERATROL, GRAPES AND RED WINE

Hundreds of plant extracts have been evaluated for anticancer qualities. One promising discovery has been resveratrol, initially identified as the active ingredient in a plant from Peru which was found to have anti-inflammatory (and therefore potentially anticancer) properties.

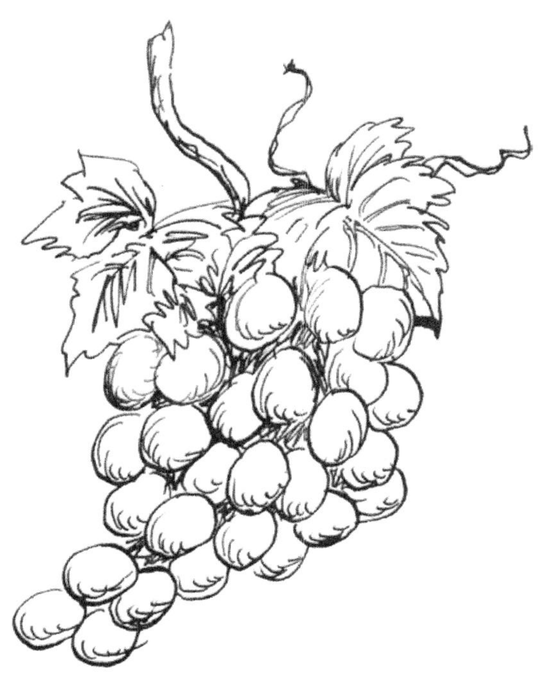

Resveratrol is quite well-known for its promotion (perhaps a little too enthusiastically) as an anti-ageing supplement because it extended the life span of yeast and fish. It is also widely used for weight loss, and to enhance endurance and energy.

Our focus is against cancer.

Evidence

Resveratrol has such an amazing array of anticancer effects that it warrants inclusion in this book, despite most of the evidence being at laboratory level.

There are small mountains of scientific papers published regarding this plant chemical, demonstrating that it blocks the proliferation of almost all cancer cell lines by a multitude of different molecular mechanisms[1-6]. Resveratrol can sensitize cancer cells to chemotherapy[7]. It is an anti-inflammatory, an antioxidant and an immune system modulator, which are all means of protection against cancer. The evidence comes mainly from cell cultures, and to a lesser extent in animals, but there have not been any human trials, apart from testing its safety[8].

Resveratrol in red wine has been postulated as a possible factor in the so-called French Paradox (reasonable health despite potentially unhealthy habits). Red wine was thought to reduce the risk of prostate cancer[9] but this has not been supported by further investigation[10,11]. However, red wine is often a poor source of resveratrol.

Resveratrol acts as a phyto-oestrogen which means that it modulates oestrogen levels, being either pro- or anti-oestrogenic depending on other factors[12]. It is probably wise for women with a history of oestrogen receptor-positive breast cancer to avoid resveratrol supplementation.

Why Should it Work?

Plants produce resveratrol in response to exposure to ultraviolet irradiation, fungi, other microbes, or other kinds of stress or injury[13]. It is a natural antibiotic and antifungal. Success against these things also lends itself to fighting cancer. This is the same principle seen with other key anticancer plants. The chemical looks after the plant and when we eat it, we receive the benefits, too.

Sources and Doses

The best known sources are red, purple and black grapes, particularly the skins and seeds, with very little resveratrol in the flesh[14]. Peeled seedless grapes will not do! Green grapes do not contain resveratrol or anthocyanins (which give the red colour). It has been said that Muscadine or Concord grapes contain the most resveratrol but this will vary depending on subtype, geographical source, etc. The use of fungicides by the farmer will result in less resveratrol because the grape plant makes more of it when exposed to fungus[14,15]. Organic grapes will be better in this regard. See p.173 for a discussion on grape types and growing regions for wine enthusiasts. Red wines from the northern hemisphere have the best resveratrol content. The

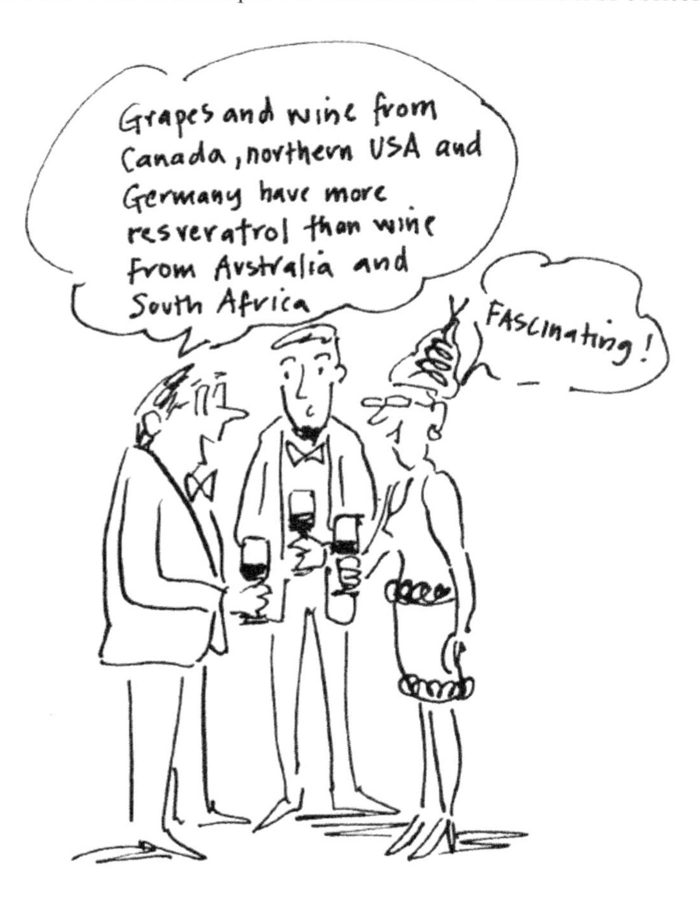

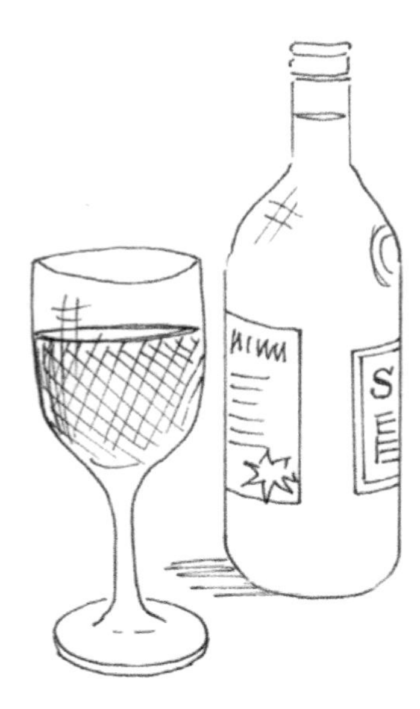

fermentation process in producing wine from grapes helps because the alcohol dissolves the resveratrol to release it from the skins and seeds. This is why there is much less resveratrol in white wine (no grape skins) and grape juice (no fermentation).

Other edible sources are peanuts (especially sprouted peanuts), mulberries, cranberries, blueberries, and jackfruit. The resveratrol content varies enormously in all these plants. Resveratrol is degraded by cooking, and also by exposure to oxygen from which it is protected by being bottled.

Supplements are available, and the dose is 50 to 250mg per day. These have mainly been promoted to the anti-ageing and weight loss groups. This dose is much higher than what can be achieved from food or wine, but such high doses may not be necessary if synergy with other beneficial food elements occurs.

Bioavailability

It is difficult to achieve high blood levels of resveratrol, and this is the subject of ongoing research. However, a very high dose may not be necessary. Surprisingly, it has been shown that low doses were more effective than high doses in preventing bowel cancers in rats[16].

What to Do?

It is tempting to justify the consumption of red wine. However, two glasses is probably not enough for a good dose of resveratrol, unless the grapes are known to be sourced from the best areas. More than two glasses is not advised because although red wine is protective, alcohol in general increases cancer risk, as well as other health problems.

Information available indicates that a good helping of grapes has as much resveratrol as a glass of wine. However, the skins would need to be chewed very well to release the nutrients. Also, where did your grapes come from? Were they sprayed? Have they been bred with thin skin or no seeds?

A supplement (up to 250mg per day) may be the best way to get some resveratrol and there are plenty of these available. If you are at high risk, this may be worthwhile. For others, grapes and the occasional glass of red wine may still be helpful. The benefits from red wine, such as a reduction in prostate cancer, may also be due to other elements working alone or synergistically with resveratrol. Women with an increased risk of breast cancer should be wary of alcohol, but if you do have a drink, choose red wine. Perhaps the resveratrol and other plant chemicals in red wine will counterbalance the cancer risk from the alcohol.

Side Effects

Resveratrol has been shown to be very safe in humans even at high doses[8]. However, it can interfere with blood clotting which means that it should be ceased prior to surgical procedures, and those on blood-thinning medication may need closer monitoring and dose adjustments.

Key Points

- Laboratory evidence shows resveratrol to be effective against cancer, but human evidence is lacking at present.
- Skins and seeds of organic dark grapes are the best source.
- Resveratrol content of red wine will depend on the grape-growing region.
- Consider a supplement if you are in a high risk group.

9. SELENIUM

Professor Edgar N Drake has written a book entitled "Selenium: Are you getting enough to reduce your risk of cancer?"[1]. It contains key information which I have utilized for parts of this chapter.

Selenium is an element present in soil. It passes to us in various foods including whole grains, nuts (especially Brazil nuts), garlic, sunflower seeds, seaweed, poultry, eggs, and seafood such as tuna, cod and oysters. However, some soils are depleted while others have high levels, so the selenium content of the above foods depends on where they come from.

Selenium is required for the proper formation and folding of dozens of proteins, including deiodinase enzymes for thyroid hormone and antioxidant enzymes.

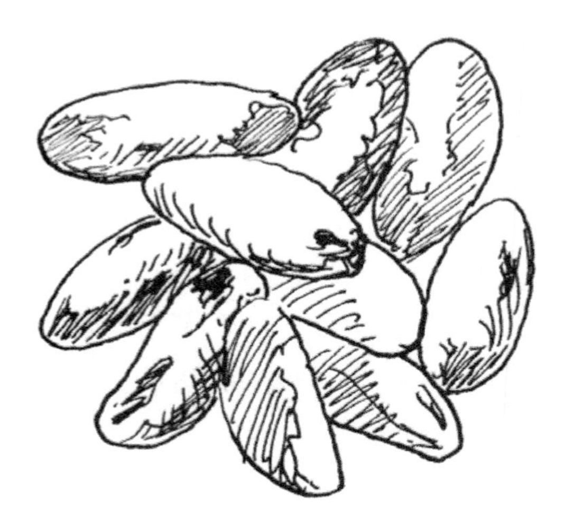

Population and Laboratory Studies

It has been known for decades that selenium in the diet relates to incidence of cancer in a community[2]. More selenium equates to less cancer, and less selenium means more cancer. Populations with a higher intake of selenium have a lower cancer death rate.

When people who are initially cancer free are followed over several years, the ones who develop cancer are the ones who had lower levels of selenium in their blood to begin with[3].

In rodent studies, animals given selenium produce far fewer cancers than the others[4].

When human cancer cells grown in the laboratory are exposed to selenium at amounts comparable to a diet from a high selenium area, about half of the cancer cells are killed[5]. Normal benign cells are unharmed.

Human Studies

The standout study, which has been virtually ignored, is the one by Clark from the University of Arizona[6]. Selenium supplementation in hundreds of trial participants was shown to greatly reduce cancer incidence. However, the validity was questioned because it was an unexpected result affecting cancer types which were not the primary subject of study. The argument goes that if you make an unintentional discovery in this way, there may be unidentified confounding (interfering) variables which you did not allow for, given that you set out to look at something different. However, this does not seem to be a good reason to totally discount this finding, when there is no other reasonable explanation.

Drake summarizes four human prevention studies from China. Selenium was shown to reduce liver cancers in two of them[7] and reduce overall deaths from cancer in another[8]. The fourth looked at oesophageal cancer and showed no difference[9], but the selenium supplement was given with zinc which may have blocked the selenium effect.

Different Forms of Selenium *(also see p.178)*

There seems to be confusion regarding which forms of selenium are most effective.

The first form of selenium is inorganic (as found in soil) including selenate and selenite, neither of which we would normally ingest with food, but can be obtained as supplements.

The second form is organic, as would be obtained from natural foods. Two of these are **selenomethionine (SM)** and **methylseleno-cysteine (MSC)**. The supplement used in Clark's study was high selenium yeast. This is known to contain mainly SM but about 20% of it is other selenium forms. In fact SM is the poorer performer against cancer, and yet it is the one used in most selenium supplements and continues to be promoted as optimal. Perplexingly, SM was the supplement used in a major study called the SELECT study[10] which was looking to see if the benefits of selenium could be duplicated (this time combined with Vitamin E). Remember, Clark did not use isolated SM but the more natural mixture of selenium forms extracted from yeast. The SELECT study was abandoned early because it was showing no benefit, and is now held up as casting doubt on selenium's role, even though they used the wrong supplement!

The best form of organic selenium seems to be MSC, which is mainly obtained from garlic grown in a selenium-rich environment. Leeks, onions and broccoli have also been used. Recently this has become available as a commercial supplement. Even so, the most readily available supplement continues to be SM. The inorganic sodium selenite is less favoured, perhaps because it is more likely to be toxic, is not a natural source for humans, and is no more effective against cancer in vivo.

Mechanism of Action

Selenium:

1. Is needed for synthesis of certain antioxidants (selenoproteins).
2. Induces apoptosis (cancer cell suicide).
3. Improves the immune system.

Of these, the apoptosis effect is probably the most important. However, it only comes into play if there is enough selenium left over after the antioxidant system has been supplied first. That is why an adequate dose is so important.

Brazil Nuts

Brazil nuts contain at least ten times more selenium than any other food and are an increasingly popular source. An average nut weighs 4g, with an average dose of selenium per nut of about 25mcg. However, it ranges very widely from just 20mcg to as high as 84mcg per nut[11].

It has been said that there is less selenium in a nut that has had its shell removed prior to sale compared with one that you shell yourself just before eating it. However, analysis of the data suggests that it depends more on the geographical origin of the nut[12]. They are not easy nuts to shell (at least in my hands).

The main factor determining the selenium content of the nut is the soil in which it is grown. Unfortunately, you will probably have trouble finding where your particular Brazil nuts come from.

How Much do I Need?

In Clark's study, the supplement was 200mcg. The diet in that population was estimated to contain about 200mcg anyway, giving a total of 400mcg.

The Recommended Daily Allowance (RDA) varies between countries from 55 to 85mcg for men and less for women and children. This is based on the amount required to generate selenoproteins. However, this is not enough for our anticancer purpose. The optimum cancer-fighting effect of selenium requires that it be in surplus to allow conversion to the active methylselenol form. A safe daily intake is in the order of 400 to 900mcg /d (much more than the RDA)[1,13]. If we allow for 200mcg already in the diet, then a supplement of 200mcg is certainly in the safe range. Most people in the UK, Australia, New Zealand, parts of Europe and parts of the USA have less than 100mcg in their diet[14], and might be better off supplementing with 300mcg if they are actively battling cancer.

Selenium is quite quickly excreted from the body, and therefore requires regular replenishment (e.g. daily).

Caution

Selenium may "thin the blood", so those on other blood-thinners like aspirin, warfarin, and clopidogrel need to be cautious. It may also reduce the effect of statins (to lower cholesterol).

Selenium overdose (especially >900mcg/d) can cause selenosis, which consists of brittle hair and nails, nausea, vomiting, and fatigue.

Supplement Advice

If you are seeking to reduce your cancer risk, consider taking extra selenium. The best food source is Brazil nuts, in which case as many as eight nuts/day may be needed to gain 200mcg of selenium. However, this may be more nuts than you want to eat, and some nuts will contain more selenium, so four nuts a day is reasonable. If your nuts unexpectedly happen to have twice as much selenium in them, you will still be well within the safe limit.

If choosing a commercial supplement, use one with methylselenocysteine (MSC) from selenium-rich garlic, which can be purchased online. If it is not available, go with selenium-rich yeast. The readily-available pure selenomethionine (SM) supplement is less likely to be beneficial.

Go nuts!

Key Points

- People living in regions with selenium-rich soil have lower rates of cancer.
- Selenium blocks cancer in the laboratory and in human studies.
- The best food source is Brazil nuts – take four to eight per day.
- The best supplement is methylselenocysteine (MSC) – take 200-300mcg per day.

Box: Magnesium

The average American diet is deficient in magnesium as a result of soil depletion (no magnesium in fertilizers), food processing (refined flour, polished rice), boiling vegetables, possibly too much dietary calcium (supplements and dairy products), and the loss of magnesium from water due to filtering or fluoride. The daily intake one hundred years ago was 500mg, but is now only about 200mg, despite the recommended intake being 300-400mg/day. Magnesium is found in many fruit and vegetables but the best dietary sources are green leafy vegetables like spinach (magnesium is in chlorophyll which gives the green colour), nuts (especially almonds, cashews, peanuts, and peanut butter), unrefined grains, lentils, beans, and bananas.

Magnesium deficiency cannot be easily diagnosed. Nearly all (99%) of the body's magnesium is inside the cells, so a blood test does not accurately reflect total levels. A red blood cell magnesium is not much better. Blood tests can be normal even when the body is deficient overall. Unless you eat a lot of vegetables, fruit and nuts, you are probably deficient, especially if you eat processed food, including refined flour products. Magnesium is depleted by excessive calcium and by alcohol.

Magnesium is a key element present in hundreds of enzyme systems, but does it have anything to do with cancer? In general terms, cells that are not functioning at their optimal level will be prone to degeneration and disease. Magnesium is needed for maintenance of electrolyte levels in cells (helps to pump sodium out and potassium in), subsequent mitochondrial energy production, acid-base balance and numerous other cellular functions. It is quite conceivable that magnesium deficiency can tip this complex balance in favour of malignancy.

A number of studies have identified an association between magnesium deficiency and colon cancer[15-18]. Low cancer rates in Egypt coincide with high dietary magnesium[19].

Magnesium helps to convert vitamin D to its active form. This is why vitamin D supplements could make a magnesium deficiency worse (uses up magnesium), and perhaps why large doses of vitamin D sometimes don't seem to work (not enough magnesium). Vitamin D protects against cancer, so indirectly magnesium deficiency could increase risk.

People at high risk of cancer or recurrence should consider supplementing with magnesium. Others can rely on dietary intake, which should be adequate if you follow the message from this book.

10. CARROTS, CAROTENE AND COLOUR

You may have heard it said that we should eat many colours, and here are some of the best ones.

What are Carotenes?

The best known carotenes are alpha-carotene, beta-carotene, and lycopene.

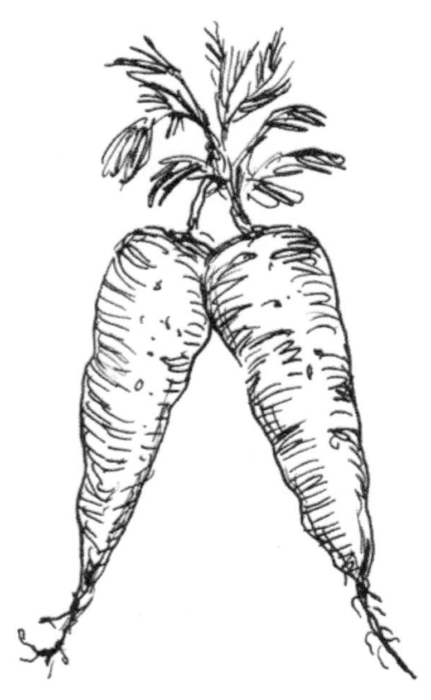

Beta-carotene is most famous for its orange or yellow colour. It is found in fruits such as pawpaw, rock melon (cantaloupes), mangoes, mandarins, oranges, and vegetables like carrots, sweet potato, pumpkin and winter squash. It is also present in green vegetables including spinach and kale, but its colour is masked by the green of chlorophyll.

Alpha-carotene is present in the same vegetables as beta-carotene above but also in peas, green beans, avocado and broccoli. Broccoli is a cruciferous vegetable and has other important anticancer chemicals.

Lycopene gives plants a vivid red colour and is best obtained from tomatoes. It is also in red carrots, red peppers, red pawpaw, goji berries and watermelons (but not in every red food. E.g. not in strawberries or cherries). Tomatoes provide much more lycopene than other sources (except a thing called gac which is not commonly eaten outside Southeast Asia).

Carotenes play a role in photosynthesis in plants and also protect the plant from excessive light damage. This protective role may be why they protect those who eat them from cancer.

Can They Stop Cancer? What do the Studies Show?

The Collaborative Breast Cancer Study compared 5,707 women who had breast cancer with those who did not. The risk of cancer was significantly lower in those who consumed food containing carotenoids, but this only applied to premenopausal women. The group who ate at least two servings per day had 17% less cancers, compared to those who had less than four servings per week[1].

The Black Women's Health Study of nearly 52,000 women showed that vegetables in general reduce ER-negative breast cancer incidence by 43%. Carrots specifically produced a 17% reduction in risk. This required at least three servings of carrots per week, compared to less than once a month[2]. (Yes, coincidentally, both studies found a risk reduction of 17%).

Lycopene Fights Prostate Cancer

Men having prostate cancer surgery were told to eat at least one meal per day with tomato sauce for three weeks before surgery.

Prostate tissue samples showed high levels of lycopene and less DNA damage[3].

Another study showed that prostate cancer risk was seen to be reduced significantly in men who had two or more servings of tomato sauce per week[4]. Some other reports have been mixed[5].

Can Carrots Cure Cancer?

Carrots and beetroot have been favourites as cancer cures in some circles (e.g. Gerson Therapy), particularly raw and juiced, and often for the purpose of detoxification. However, there is less support for carrots (compared to some other vegetables) as a major anticancer food in scientific publications. There are plenty of anecdotal reports (individual experiences) of people whose cancer went away after drinking copious amounts of carrot juice, but that kind of evidence is not very reliable. It would seem unwise to focus on carrots as the mainstay of an anticancer program.

Beets may not beat it on their own, either. There is very little in the published research about beetroot and its red/purple pigment betacyanin, apart from cancer cure reports from the 1950s[6], and some more recent rat studies. Beetroots are a good source of fibre which is certainly beneficial. Some people will develop red urine which in itself is harmless, but excessive beetroot should be avoided in those prone to kidney stones, particularly in the massive doses that have been advocated.

How do Carotenoids Work? - Mechanism of Action *(see p.179)*

Carotenes work as antioxidants and by directly blocking cancer growth via vitamin A production. Lycopene blocks IGF (a growth factor) and inhibits angiogenesis.

What Should I Eat and How Much?

Eat a wide array of colours. The presence of many colours indicates a variety of complementary plant pigments (carotenes and others), many of which work against cancer. The preservation of bright colour indicates well preserved produce and healthy preparation (not over-cooked). Nearly every plant has some anticancer properties because all plants need to protect themselves against

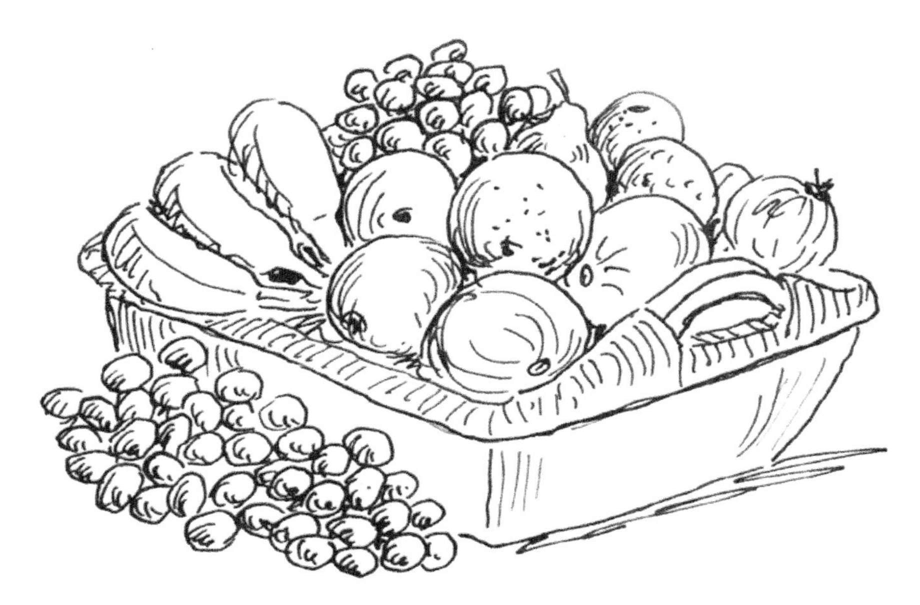

microbes, cell damage from internal chemical reactions, or environmental injury.

Eating a diversity of plants can reduce cancer risk. It has been reported that lung cancer risk in smokers was affected more by variety than quantity. Most benefit was shown when more of eight particular types were eaten, with each additional type reducing risk by a further 4%. The eight subgroups of vegetables used were: leafy vegetables, fruiting vegetables, root vegetables, cabbages, mushrooms, grain and pod vegetables, onion and garlic, and stalk vegetables[7]. This paper also describes several other studies which reported that a greater variety in diet, especially of fruit and vegetables, reduces the incidence of other cancers as well.

There are a number of explanations as to why diversity beats quantity. It could be that for a certain individual, a particular element is needed, and it is more likely to be obtained if the diet is wide. Agricultural sources vary and some are better quality than others. Perhaps some fruit and vegetable subgroups are being prepared or cooked more appropriately. It is likely that synergy between a number of phytochemicals is more powerful than larger quantities of a single one. All of the above reasons are probably valid.

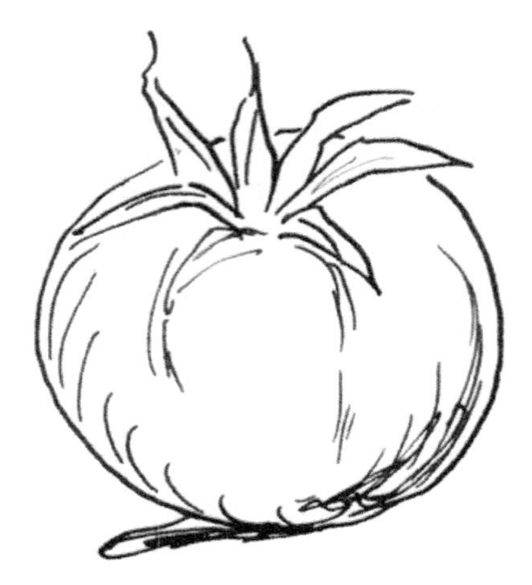

Tomatoes

Ripe tomatoes are best - more red equals more lycopene[8]. In contrast to other foods (which are better if raw or lightly cooked), cooking and processing tomatoes into juice or sauce is the way to go. This actually increases the concentration and bioavailability of lycopene[9]. It is well absorbed when cooked and eaten with oil-rich food such as Italian food because it is fat soluble[10]. All carotenes are absorbed better if eaten with avocado (such as tomato salsa with guacamole), presumably due to the avocado oil[11]. If you are at increased risk of prostate cancer, tomatoes offer a defensive strategy.

Even just two meals a week with tomato paste or sauce is helpful, but you could have it every day. Try to avoid the ones with too much added sugar or salt.

Carrots

Risk reduction for breast cancer (all types) required two carrots per day in one major study, whereas another needed three per week but only protected against one cancer subtype.

Should carrots be raw or cooked? Raw carrots are effective, provided they are very well chewed, otherwise most of the beta-carotene is not released. Juicing or pulping will release more nutrients. Cooking also releases beta-carotene from carrots by softening the cell walls[12]. Nutrients are said to be more concentrated under the skin[13], so it is probably best not to peel them, but they should be washed.

Beta-carotene gives people an orange hue to their skin ("carotenaemia"), especially affecting the palms and the face, if taken in large amounts. This won't hurt you, but can become quite a feature!

Key Points

- Carotenoids from carrots and other orange or yellow fruit and vegetables, are linked to lower rates of breast cancer.
- Lycopene, the red pigment in tomatoes, reduces prostate cancer risk.
- Tomatoes are most effective when ripe, cooked, and consumed in an oil-rich meal.
- Protection from cancer can be achieved by having two meals per week with tomato sauce or paste, and by eating two carrots per day (or even three times per week).

Other Key Players

These did not quite make it into the top ten, either because the evidence is not as strong, information is less abundant, or research is in an earlier phase. However, they should be considered as part of the team.

On the other hand, we need to know about the players that we don't want on the field, and these are discussed here, too.

11. PROBIOTICS

The term probiotics refers to beneficial colonic bacteria. Probiotics do not feature much in cancer research, but there is enough information to make it worth mentioning.

The key probiotics are Lactobacillus (various species, including acidophilus, helveticus, casei), and Bifidobacterium. They are termed lactic acid bacilli (LAB) because they produce lactic acid by

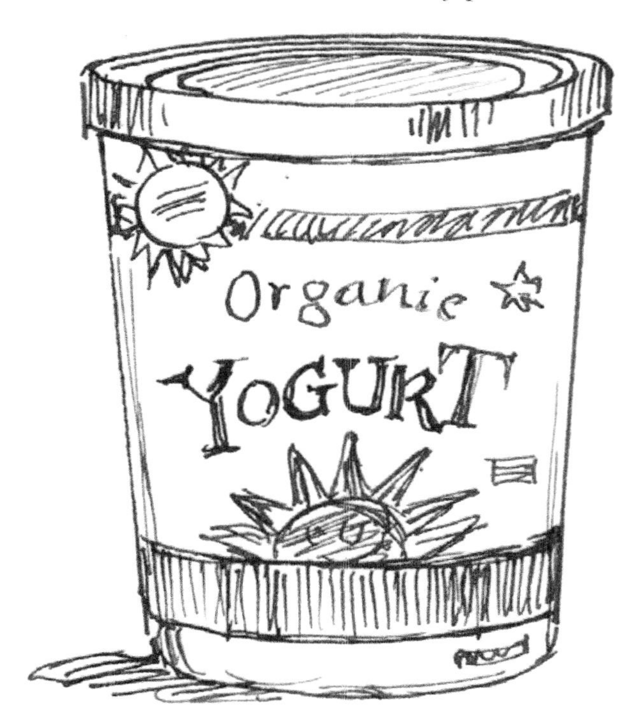

fermenting lactose. The acidity gives fermented dairy products a tart taste, and is unfavourable for the growth of harmful bacteria in the bowel.

Most of the evidence for probiotics has been in animals and other laboratory work, as well as some population studies. There is some indirect evidence in humans and a few other noteworthy studies. See p.181.

We naturally have billions of beneficial bacteria in our large bowel, but when these become depleted, not only do we lose their direct favourable functions, but their loss allows unhealthy bacteria to flourish, leading to increased cancer risk. The depletion of the good bacteria may occur because we don't eat enough of the food that nourishes them (prebiotics). Antibiotics certainly destroy intestinal bacteria, and are linked to increased breast cancer risk[1]. Mercury exposure alters gut bacteria[2,3].

Mechanism of Action *(see p.182)*

The gut lumen carries a burden of toxic substances such as bile acids, amines, sulphates, bacterial toxins, and excreted metabolic waste. Beneficial bacteria are able to negate a number of these. For example, they bind oestrogen, nitrosamines, heavy metals and other potential carcinogens, removing them from the gut before they can cause damage.

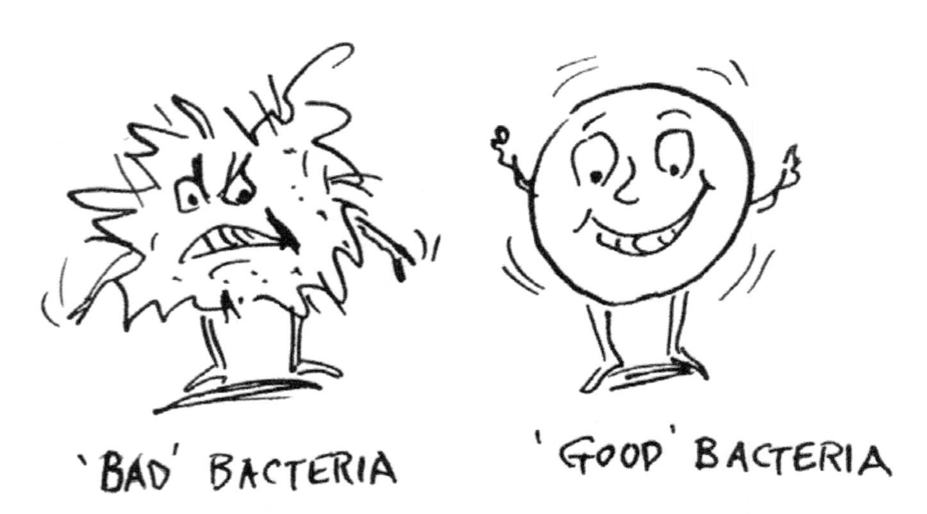

They suppress bad bacteria and putrefactive organisms like yeasts, by competing with them for nutrients, or by directly consuming them, thus preventing their production of carcinogens.

Beneficial bacteria produce anticancer fatty acids such as butyrate and CLA.

They also play an increasingly recognized role in the immune system.

What Can You Do?

Take probiotics and/or prebiotics as supplements or as food.

Once again, we aim to achieve our goal with real food when possible, and there are distinct advantages of food over supplements[4]. There is much yet to be discovered in this field, and supplements may miss the mark because we don't know enough about what is required for maximal effect. Food sources, on the other hand, bring a complex mixture of nutrients (and in this case, bacteria) with both known and unknown benefits. Unlike fermented foods, supplements are more limited in number and type of bacteria, which are further threatened by transport and storage. They also cost more.

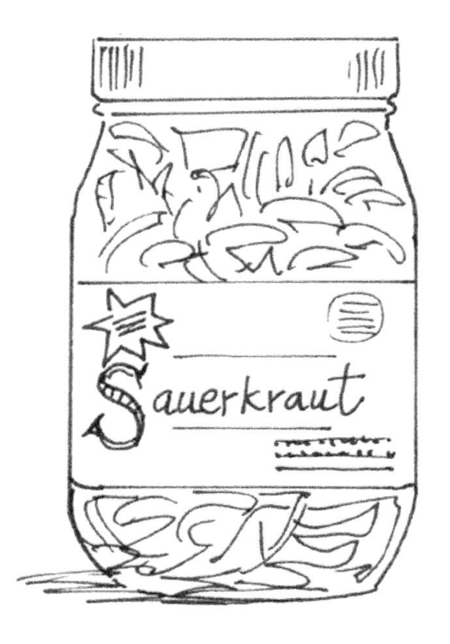

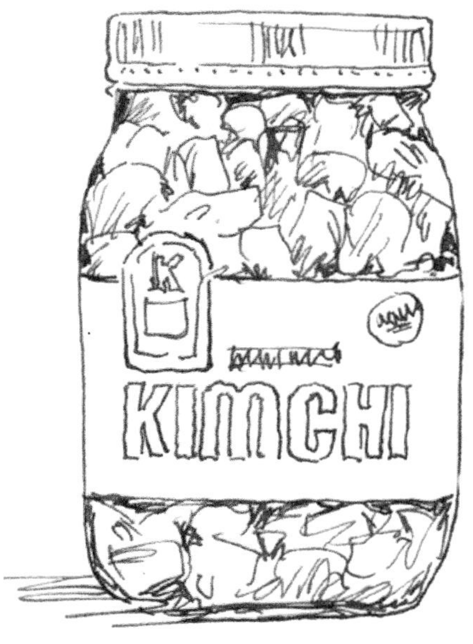

Supplements

There are many supplements to choose from. Look for one with a high count of bacteria, and with bacteria of more than one or two species from the list above. Seek a reputable brand because inferior ones will have less reliable preservation of bacteria in the capsule. Soil-based organisms are not recommended because they have the potential to overgrow and become pathogenic (i.e. cause disease).

Prebiotics

More recently recognized, prebiotics are foods that stimulate the growth of beneficial bacteria. Prebiotics have a similar end result to probiotics because they are feeding the good bacteria that are already there.

The list includes garlic, onions, leeks, bananas, agave, asparagus, Jerusalem artichokes, dandelion greens, and chicory root[5]. These last two are said to be the best but are not widely consumed in large amounts, whereas onions and bananas have smaller concentrations but are eaten in larger volumes. Beans, pulses and oats are less potent sources. Cooking reduces the prebiotic content to some extent.

Real Food Probiotics

Include natural sources such as yoghurt and fermented vegetables as a regular part of your diet. Probiotics do not cause a permanent increase in bacterial numbers, so they need to be consumed regularly.

Yoghurt has to be natural yoghurt, not processed, pasteurized, flavoured and full of sugar. The bacteria types should be listed on the container. It is easy to make your own yoghurt, but the bacterial count will not be as high as the ones produced commercially.

Other fermented (or cultured) food includes sauerkraut, kimchi, kefir, aged cheeses, kombucha, pickled fruits, etc. These are all traditional foods with reputations as health-giving. Commercially available versions may have been pasteurized to improve shelf life, but this obviously kills any beneficial bacteria, and our purpose is defeated. The same applies to cheeses.

Therefore, you either need to find a supplier of the genuine article or make it yourself. This is definitely worth trying and apparently not difficult. For example, making sauerkraut involves shredding the vegetables and covering for several days at the right temperature, often with a starter culture added. Happy fermenting!

Key Points

- Probiotics are strains of bacteria that live in the large bowel and help to prevent cancer.
- They remove toxins from material in the bowel, suppress harmful microbes, and produce anticancer butyrate.
- Garlic, onions, leeks, bananas, asparagus and Jerusalem artichokes stimulate the growth of beneficial bacteria.
- Fermented foods such as yoghurt and sauerkraut, are good sources of probiotics.
- Consider exploring exotic sources such as kefir, kimchi, kombucha and miso soup.
- Supplements need to be good quality, preferably with more than one type of bacteria and with high bacteria counts.

12. FIBRE

It is generally agreed that high dietary fibre protects against colorectal cancer[1], and it has been postulated (but not proven) that other cancers may be reduced as well.

Why would fibre work against cancer?

There are a number of possible reasons.

1. Fibre adds bulk to stools, which moves them through the bowel faster. This reduces the time in which potential cancer-producing toxins are in contact with the bowel lining.
2. The bulky stool will dilute carcinogens, and the fibre itself binds to certain carcinogens, removing them with the stool.
3. Fermentation of fibre by beneficial bacteria produces a short-chain fatty acid called butyrate, which inhibits cancer cells[2,3]. The quantity of butyrate-producing bacteria is greater in the bowels of high fibre diet people compared to those with low fibre diets[4].
4. Fibre slows down the absorption of sugar, stabilizing blood sugar and insulin levels. Elevated insulin and IGF (insulin-like growth factor) can potentially stimulate cancer growth[5,6].
5. Fibre prevents constipation which possibly increases breast cancer risk. Women who have only two bowel motions per week are more likely to have abnormal (dysplastic) cells in breast duct fluid[7]. This could be because constipation may inhibit bacterial metabolism of oestrogen.
6. Fibre eaters are less likely to be obese. Diets with high fibre (more fruit and vegetables, less meat, less processed carbohydrate)

are usually associated with a lean figure. If you are eating food with fibre, you won't be eating fattening food. High fibre food requires more chewing and a greater feeling of fullness, leading to earlier satiety, and lower caloric intake. On the other hand, obesity carries a high cancer risk.

Of course, foods that are high in fibre (fruit and vegetables) will lower cancer risk by other means as well.

Fibre supplements, such as wheat bran and psyllium husk (ispaghula), do not seem to be protective[8], and may actually increase the risk of precancerous bowel polyps and recurrence of polyps[9]. As well as binding and removing toxins, fibre can bind and negate beneficial nutrients and minerals. Fibre supplements with inadequate fluid intake may be counterproductive by causing constipation. It is unnecessary (and possibly detrimental) to take fibre as a supplement.

Enough fibre can be obtained from a healthy plant-based diet which also provides a broad spectrum of other anticancer nutrients.

13. IODINE

Some writers are convinced that iodine has an important role to play against cancer[1,2], while others are less certain.

The case for iodine as a cancer preventer or controller is begun here and more evidence is presented on p.184.

1. There is an association between iodine deficiency and breast cancer. Populations that consume more iodine have less breast cancer, and those that have less iodine have more breast cancer. People who suffer with autoimmune thyroid disease or goitre (thyroid enlargement, often due to iodine deficiency) have two to three times the incidence of breast cancer compared with those with normal thyroids[3]. Conversely, breast cancer patients are much more likely to have some form of thyroid disease[4].

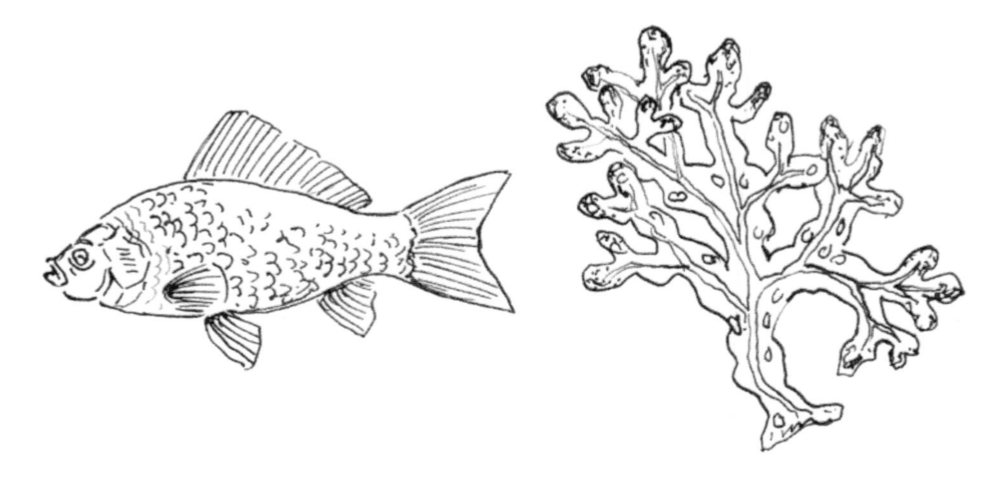

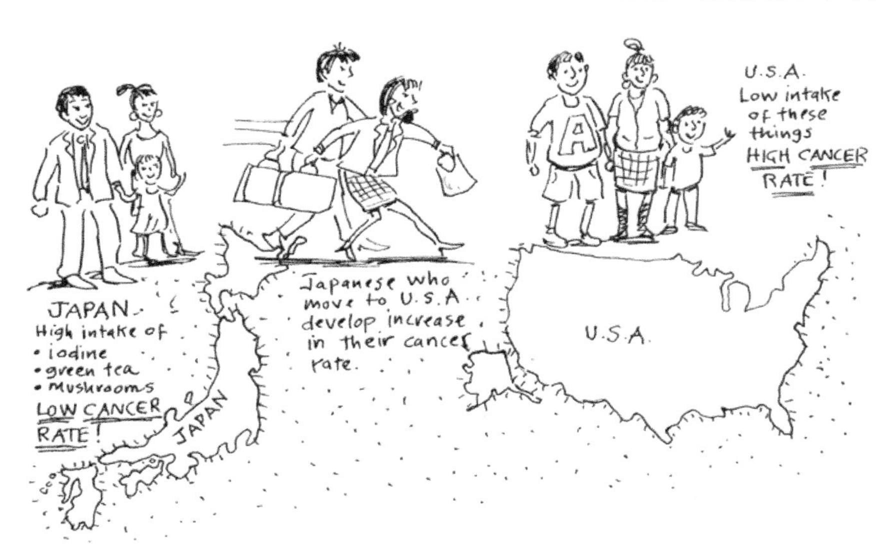

In Japan, the average intake of iodine is about 14mg per day (mainly in the form of seaweed), compared to less than 1mg in the West. The Japanese have a low incidence of cancer of the breast and prostate. This is clouded by the fact that the Japanese also consume a lot of vegetables and green tea which will also reduce cancer risk. The Japanese mortality rate from breast cancer is 7 per 100,000 people, compared to UK and USA at 28 and 22 per 100,000, respectively. However, the rates go up in Japanese who emigrate to the West[5].

In Iceland, fishmeal has been traditionally fed to dairy cattle, resulting in high iodine levels in milk. When the fishmeal quantities were reduced to comply with international standards, the incidence of breast cancer went up tenfold[2].

In Spain, regions with low iodine intake have the highest breast cancer mortality[6].

2. In experiments with rats, cancers are produced by exposing them to carcinogens. The rats that are given iodine are less likely to develop the tumours[7].
3. Iodine reduces the responsiveness of genes to oestrogen[8], and has a number of other anti-oestrogenic effects[9].
4. Iodine causes apoptosis (programmed cell death). Rats that were growing three different breast cancer cell lines were given

a Mekabu (seaweed) solution in drinking water. Thereafter, the cancer cells were observed to have a high rate of apoptosis, and the effect was greater than that of 5-FU (a common cancer chemotherapy agent)[10].

5. Iodine deficiency is linked to fibrocystic change (FCC) in the breast, and thus appears to enhance the sensitivity of mammary tissue to oestrogen (which is what causes breast hyperplasia). In rats, lack of iodine is seen to produce breast changes equivalent to human FCC[11]. In humans, iodine supplements at 6mg/day for six months will reduce FCC (including breast pain and benign lumpiness) in at least 50% of sufferers[12]. Brown sea algae (a source of iodine) reduced breast pain and nodularity in 94%[13].

   Benign breast disease is said to be a precursor for cancer, but it should be pointed out that this is really only the case when atypia is present (abnormal cells) which is only in the minority of FCC[14]. The idea is that because so many women (probably the majority) have some degree of FCC, there will be a significant number with atypia amongst them. Therefore if all the FCC could be treated with iodine, at least some of the atypia (and breast cancer risk) could be prevented.

How Can We Apply this Information?

Although some may dispute that there is enough evidence for iodine against cancer, we should still avoid iodine deficiency for other reasons anyway. If I had cancer, or was at increased risk, or just wanted to apply good preventative measures, I would ensure good iodine levels.

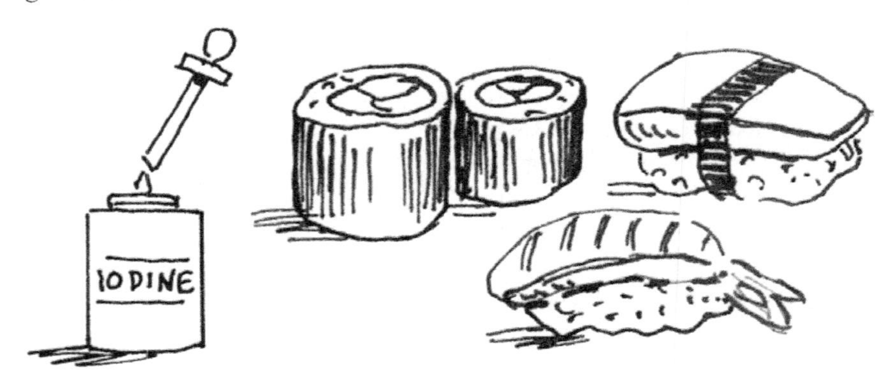

There are definite regions of iodine deficiency in Australia, despite iodine being added to salt, and more recently to bread. Many of my breast and thyroid patients are clearly deficient when formally tested by a 24 hour urinary iodine measurement. Dietary iodine can be increased through sources such as fish and seaweed. Too much fish carries a mercury risk. Seaweed is an excellent source, taken for example as sushi or by using dried seaweed sheets in cooking or snacks. Kelp supplements are available in tablet form.

Alternatively, a specific iodine supplement can be used such as Lugol's iodine solution. One drop per day gives about 3mg (depending on the dropper) which is way above (20 times) the recommended amount of 150mcg, but a fraction (about a quarter) of the average Japanese daily intake. There is very little danger in having this much iodine. Any excess will be excreted in the urine. However, the occasional person is very sensitive to it, in which case it could actually block thyroid function, resulting in an underactive thyroid. This is easily corrected by stopping the iodine. Also, in people who have a nodular or enlarged thyroid, extra iodine may cause the thyroid to become overactive. Therefore, before using iodine drops, you should have your doctor assess your thyroid for nodules, and have your thyroid hormone levels (TFTs) checked. The TFTs need to be re-checked several weeks after starting the iodine.

When you are fighting cancer, you don't want to be deficient in any dietary components. If you eat a western diet, you probably lack iodine. Iodine supplementation may help with headaches, fatigue, thyroid conditions, and breast lumps or densities (making mammograms more accurate), as well as helping to prevent cancer.

Key Points

- There is evidence that iodine has a role against cancer.
- Iodine deficiency is actually quite common, even in western countries.
- Sources include fish and seaweed, such as in seaweed salads, sushi or dried seaweed sheets.
- Supplements are available as iodine drops (or tablets in some countries) or kelp capsules.
- If you decide to take a supplement, have your thyroid assessed by your doctor, before and after commencement.

14. EVERYDAY SUPERFOODS EVERY DAY

You may have seen the term "superfoods" bandied about quite a bit. It implies that common foods are inadequate, and that we must seek something more powerful.

New or re-discovered superfoods seem to be appearing all the time, most being rather obscure or from remote locations. They come with claims for health benefits but usually without a great deal of evidence. Examples include acai berries (from a South American palm), goji berries (Himalayan), noni juice (Polynesian), chlorella (green algae from the ocean), spirulina (cyanobacteria from tropical lakes), maca (a root from the Andes), camu camu (fruit from the Amazon), and Kakadu plum (bush tucker from Australia). Generally

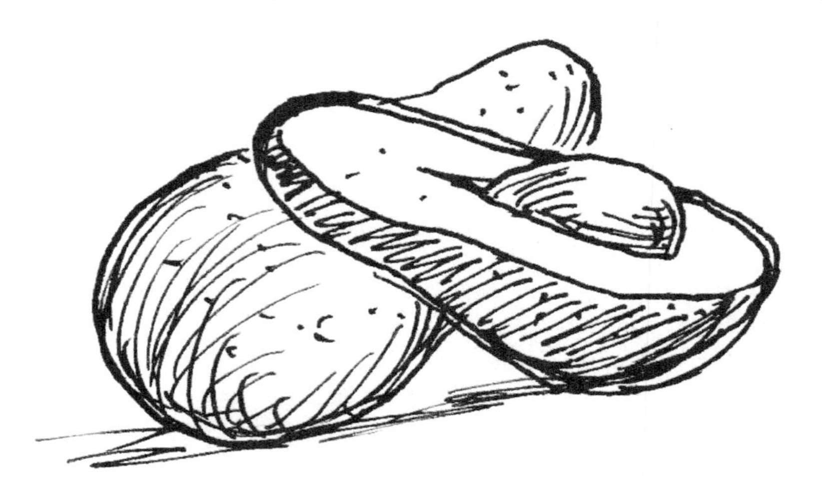

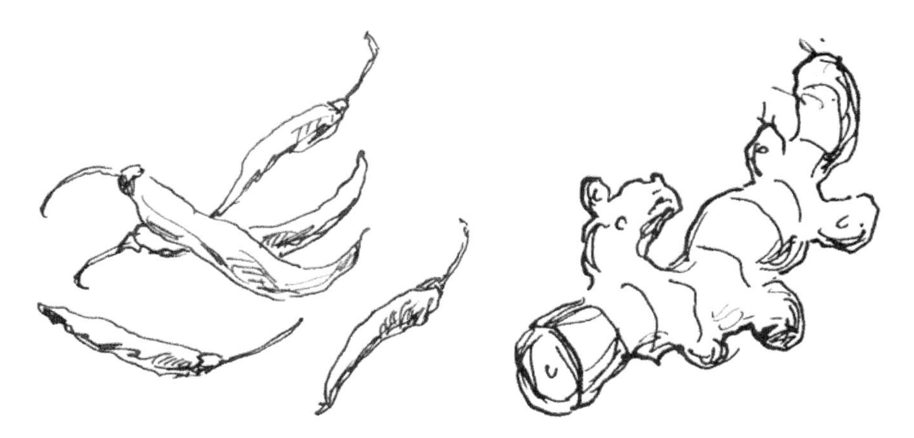

these are quite expensive, and have not been subjected to enough study to know how good they really are. I expect that many of these foods are beneficial, but it may be because they are from areas where soils (or oceans) have not been depleted of key nutrients, or that they have been farmed or harvested without chemicals or processing. On the other hand, some are only in supplement form, may not be very pure, and could be marketed by those wanting to take advantage of anxious consumers who are willing to pay for the hope of a cure.

Do we really need to seek out "superfoods"? What about everyday items? What about apples and oranges?

Fresh, locally grown common items have been extensively studied, have been shown to be protective, and are easily obtainable and affordable. By all means, eat superfoods if you want, but don't miss what is right under your nose.

I have been amazed to find how many fruits and vegetables possess anticancer activity. Perhaps they all do to some extent. Research keeps uncovering more beneficial foods in the form of unprocessed plants. This is what we would expect if we accept the principle that plants produce chemistry to protect themselves, and the same chemistry protects us when we ingest them. The preceding chapters focus on the top anticancer foods or food categories based on what is currently known, but remember that variety is probably as important as quantity, and many other fruits and vegetables have amazing qualities.

So, back to apples and oranges as our everyday examples.

Apples

Apples are extremely nutritious, containing vitamins, minerals, fibre, and many types of phytochemicals including antioxidants[1]. These constituents provide cancer protection via multiple mechanisms[2,3]. For example, APE (apple peel extract) slows the growth of cancer cells in the laboratory. It leads to production of a tumour suppressor protein called maspin which prevents cancer cell invasion and metastasis[4].

The dose of apples that blocks cancer in rats can be achieved in a human by eating just one apple a day, but the effect increases with the dose[5,6]. Many nutrients are more concentrated in the peel than the flesh, so the peel should be eaten. Variation in skin colour indicates variation in nutrients. Eating different types of apples ensures a broad exposure, with a greater chance of getting the ones that you need. Bruised apples won't be as good because there has been oxidation, causing destruction of the plant chemicals. Storage does not have negative effects[1], but processing does. For example, commercial apple juice is clear because all the best nutrients have been removed to stop the juice looking brown and cloudy.

Oranges

Oranges contains an abundance of well-known anticancer phytochemicals including carotenoids, vitamin C, and quercetin, as well as the lesser known naringenin and limonene[7].

Laboratory work shows that most citrus fruits (oranges, tangerines, limes, lemons) do block cancers. Grapefruit reports are mixed[8]. A review of available research on citrus identified 48 human studies that showed a significant protective effect against cancer, with cancer of the oesophagus and stomach the most convincing[9]. With regard to breast cancer, over 300 studies were narrowed down to the 6 most reliable. These showed breast cancer to be reduced by 10% overall, with three of them showing a 30% reduction for those eating the most citrus fruit[10].

Whole oranges are better than juice alone. The pith contributes fibre, vitamin C and phytochemicals. So don't throw out all the pith – leave a bit on the orange when you peel it, but chew it well. If you drink juice, freshly squeezed is preferred, as are juices containing some pulp. Cancer protection seems to be achievable from just half an orange per day[10,11].

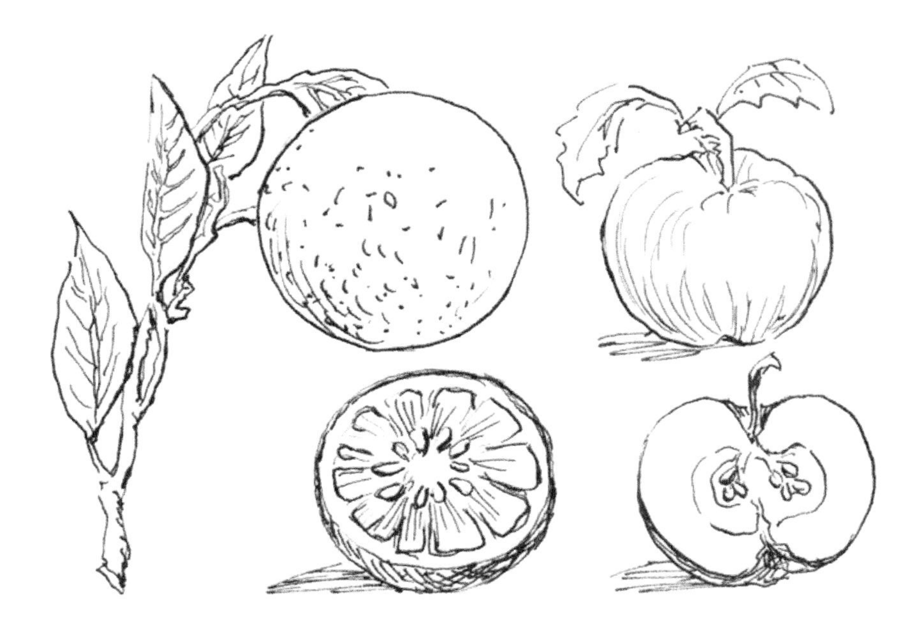

Everyday Superfoods

If apples or oranges were discovered for the first time tomorrow in a remote hidden valley, we would be running around saying what amazing superfoods they were. A lot of the plants we eat today are like that. Over many generations, we have introduced the best fruit

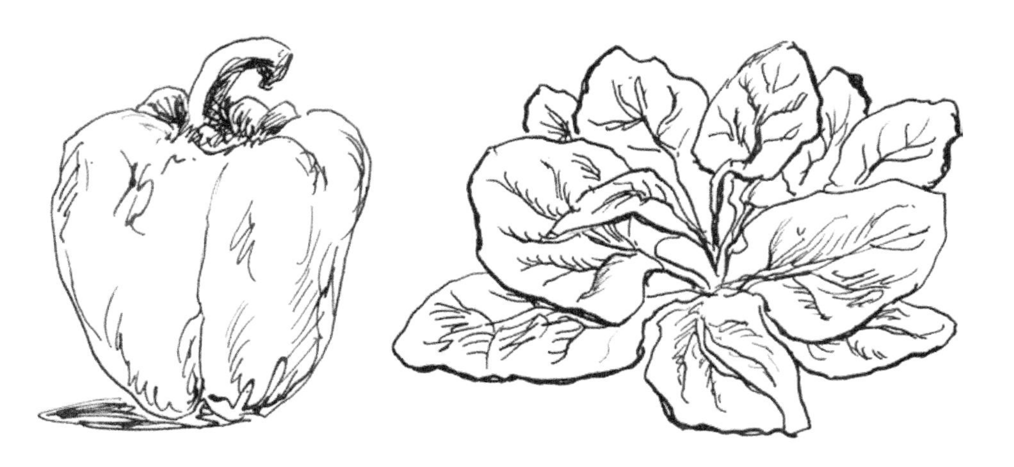

and vegetables from all over the world to our own cultures. The problem is that we just don't eat them as much as we should.

Other common plant foods with anticancer effects backed by research include:

- Pomegranate
- Pawpaw
- Pineapple
- Avocado
- Spinach
- Peppers and chillies
- Legumes (peas, beans, green beans)
- Ginger
- Many kinds of herbs and spices

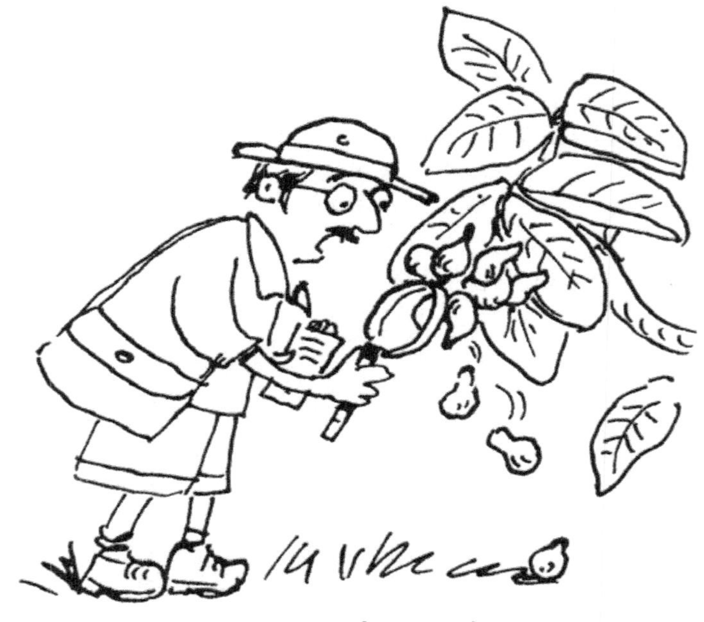

Kakadu plums - Searching for the ultimate superfood, but some everyday foods are super.

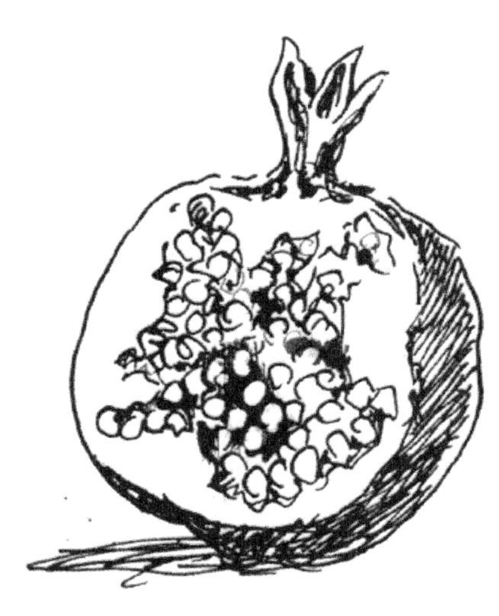

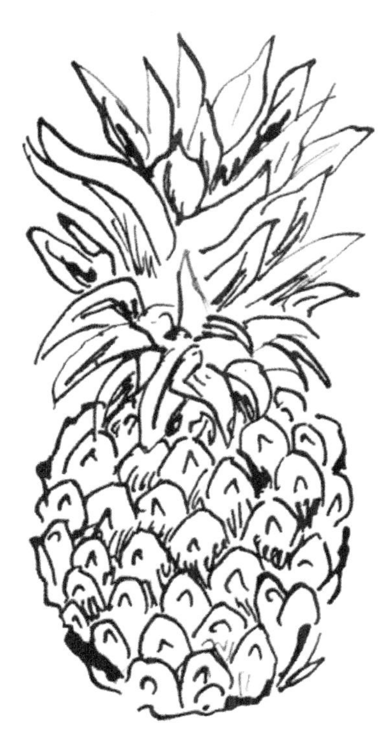

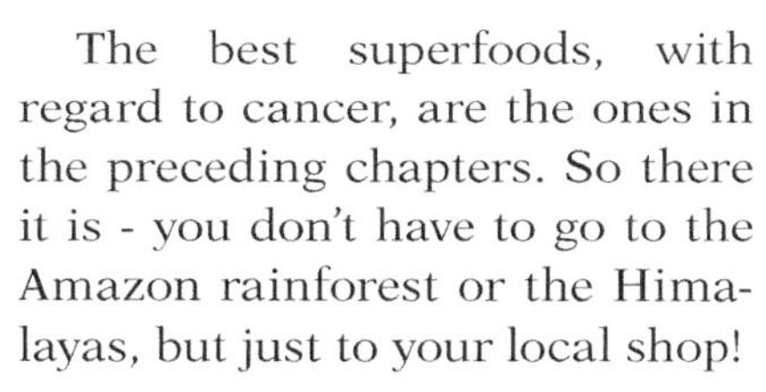

The best superfoods, with regard to cancer, are the ones in the preceding chapters. So there it is - you don't have to go to the Amazon rainforest or the Himalayas, but just to your local shop!

Key Points

- So-called superfoods are probably very beneficial, but have not been studied much, and can be expensive.
- "Everyday superfoods" include apples, oranges, pomegranates, pawpaw, pineapple, avocado, spinach, peppers, chillies, legumes (peas, beans, green beans), ginger and many herbs and spices.
- Just one apple (with peel) or an orange per day will provide an anticancer effect.

15. WHAT YOU CAN DO WITHOUT

I think most people already know what is not good for them, and I really wanted to focus this book on the positive side of food - the foods which work against cancer. However, I must also mention the foods which increase cancer risk. Sorry! They form part of the environment to which we are exposed, and this is a part that we can actually control.

The chapter contains information on alcohol, meat, and sugar, as well as obesity. These have all received the media spotlight at times, usually triggered when a journalist trips over a research paper on the subject. This chapter looks at some key medical journal articles that were picked up and aired by the media in the last year or two. Regrettably, yesterday's news goes in the bin, and becomes "out of sight, out of mind". The point is that when you see "bad" food, don't just think heart disease and waistline, but ask what it is doing to your cancer risk. These few review articles are merely a small sample of the copious amount of research on these risk factors.

Lifestyle

Medical Journal of Australia, Mar 2012 "....cancers preventable by better diet...."[1]

This article pointed out that at least 90% of cancers are due to lifestyle and environment. It showed that the habits of Australians are worsening. The percentage of sedentary Aussies has moved up to 35%, those with harmful alcohol use went up to 12%, and the overweight percentage was over 60%! This is typical of most Western countries. Less than 10% eat the recommended five serves of vegetables per day, and healthy food is becoming more expensive.

Alcohol

Journal of the American Medical Association, Nov 2011 "Moderate alcohol.. and breast cancer risk"[2]

This article concluded that moderate alcohol consumption during adult life increases breast cancer risk. About 75,000 women were followed for 20 years, during which time about 7,700 breast cancers were diagnosed (roughly 10% of the group). The alcohol drinkers were compared to non-drinkers. One drink per day increased risk by 15%, and the risk kept going up with each additional drink. Overall, the statistics indicated that each drink per day increased cancer risk by 10%, to the point where risk was increased 50% for those having more than three drinks per day.

That sounds quite frightening, doesn't it? However, statistics can be tricky. The risk discussed is what we call "relative risk". You can see that altogether about 10% of the group developed breast cancer (7,700 out of 75,000) which gives an "absolute risk" of 10%. If we increase the relative risk of cancer by 10%, it is actually 10% of the baseline 10% which is a 1% absolute increase, bringing that person's new risk to 11% (this is not precise because the increased risk is being compared to the non-drinkers, not the group average, but the point is that "relative risk" can make the difference seem bigger than it actually is).

It is important to know that a small amount of alcohol is beneficial in conferring some protection against heart disease. In the West, breast cancer causes the deaths of 1 in 25 women. Heart disease causes 1 in 3 deaths. If your breast cancer risk is low and your heart risk is high (family history, etc), then one or two drinks might not be a bad idea. For those who have had breast cancer or are at high risk, it makes sense to limit alcohol. Remember, the study looked at average daily consumption over decades - one extra drink every day for 20 years! I expect that many of you will have a drink every day, in which case your cancer risk will go up (a few percent). However, if you want to drink alcohol every now and then, or at social events, the risk is probably negligible.

What Does Alcohol Have to do With Cancer?

There are a number of possible mechanisms. It can damage tissue directly, e.g. the lining of the mouth and throat. It results in production of the carcinogen acetaldehyde in the bowel. It reduces levels of folate and magnesium, which can lead to increased cancer risk. It can raise oestrogen levels by increasing aromatase, decreasing liver metabolism of oestrogen, and enhancing oestrogen receptors.

Meat

Archives of Internal Medicine, 2012 "Red meat consumption and mortality"[3]

This paper reported on 34,000 men and 84,000 women, followed over 22 years. Deaths from cancer were recorded. The focus was on their intake of meat, and a distinction was made between unprocessed and processed meat. A serve of unprocessed meat was 80g, and a serve of processed meat was one hot dog or two slices of bacon. It was found that one serving per day of unprocessed red meat gave a 10% increased risk of dying from cancer, and the risk increased a further 10% for each additional serving per day. For processed meat, the risk increase was even higher at 16%.

Once again, this is a relative risk. The overall cancer death rate was 5% for the study group (adjusted for other risk factors), so the absolute risk increase from processed meat was 16% of 5%, which is 0.8% (similar to the increased risk from each extra drink of alcohol).

This particular study found that white meat (chicken and fish) did not increase cancer risk.

Why Would Meat Increase the Risk of Cancer?

Clearly, processing is a bad thing[4]. Processed meat often has N-nitroso compounds, formed from nitrite which is added as a preservative, and to give it a red colour and a certain flavour. High temperature cooking produces heterocyclic amines and polcyclic aromatic hydrocarbons. All these things are carcinogenic in the laboratory. For unprocessed red meat, there will be different risks for grain fed (bad) and grass fed (better), and with regard to how it is prepared.

Iron in red meat may cause oxidative damage to cells. High meat consumption is associated with an early onset of menstruation[5], which is a risk factor for breast cancer. Furthermore, meat may take the place of beneficial foods such as vegetables.

Sugar and Refined White Flour

"Sugar: The Bitter Truth" by Robert Lustig, on YouTube[6]*, and "Sweet Poison" by David Gillespie*[7]

Sugar has received much-deserved criticism in popular media hits such as these. It is implicated in several health issues, with cancer now being one of them.

There has been a startling rise in the per capita consumption of sugar over the last 70 years. One commentator has pointed out that "White table sugar, white flours, and refined baked goods with corn syrup and multiple additives are not health foods". What a surprise! It would have been natural in a primitive or hunter-gatherer situation to target high calorie food sources because food was relatively scarce. Today, we have sugary food all around us, cheaply available, and heavily marketed. However, the fact that so many others are eating and drinking it to excess, and you can get "2-for-1", does not mean you have to participate.

You have probably heard the remark "cancer feeds on sugar". It is certainly true that cancers have high metabolic demands for which they utilize sugar. This is demonstrated on PET (positron emission tomography) scans which are used to detect cancer. For these scans, the patient is injected with FDG. The G stands for glucose. The images show bright spots where the glucose has accumulated in cancer because the cancer cells take up the sugar much more strongly than do normal body cells.

Nevertheless, it is not as simple as the idea that we feed cancer with sugar, because our body regulates blood sugar levels within a certain range by secreting insulin. Recent research indicates that calorie restriction can inhibit cancer growth[8]. Foods with a high GI (glycaemic index) and high GL (glycaemic load) lead to cancer growth in lab mice, and these foods are associated with an increased risk of cancers of the breast, ovary, colon and thyroid in human population studies[9-12].

However, perhaps more importantly, high sugar intake leads to the problems of weight gain and diabetes, both of which are strongly linked to cancer[13]. They result in insulin resistance, in which normal cells no longer respond to insulin adequately. This leads us to compensate by secreting more insulin which, along with insulin-like growth factor (IGF), promotes tumour growth[14-16]. Metformin is a diabetic medication that improves insulin sensitivity and lowers insulin levels. It has been shown to have anticancer effects[17].

There are widely differing opinions about the sugars in fruit. There are so many anticancer phytochemicals in fruit that I would encourage you to keep eating sensible quantities of it, providing it is not processed. The fibre and protein in fruit slow the absorption of sugar so that insulin problems are unlikely to arise. The sugar to avoid is that added to tea, coffee, or breakfast cereal, as well as any processed food with high sugar content like soft drinks, sweets, chocolate bars, "low-fat" treats, etc. Anything made with refined white flour is also a problem because it is rapidly converted to sugar. Excessive carbohydrates are a major cause of obesity, despite being "99% fat free"!

Obesity

Oncology, Oct 2011 "Obesity and breast cancer"[18]

This paper first quotes an old study which showed that obesity at the time of diagnosis of breast cancer resulted in a lower five year survival (56% compared to 80% if lean). It later cites a recent meta-analysis (combined results of a number of studies) confirming the association, with significantly higher rates of cancer recurrences and cancer deaths among the obese[19,20]. But can we make a difference by losing weight after the diagnosis of cancer has been made? There is some inconsistency in findings, but one study showed weight gain after diagnosis was associated with more recurrences. Another showed weight loss resulted in fewer recurrences.

In the USA, more than 120,000 cases of cancer per year are linked to excess body fat[21]. There is no doubt that obesity is a significant cancer risk factor.

Why Would Obesity Increase Cancer Risk?

Obesity causes higher oestrogen levels because it is produced by the aromatase enzyme in peripheral fat. Abdominal fat is associated with higher insulin levels and with inflammation which are both linked to cancer. Leptin and adiponectin are produced in fat cells. They affect insulin sensitivity and stimulate breast cancer cells.

Dairy

This is a controversial area. In "The China Study", Colin Campbell convincingly showed that the casein protein in milk caused cancers to grow rampantly in animals[22]. Cancer survivor, Professor Jane Plant is convinced that dairy introduces a huge cancer risk[23]. She points out that substances in the blood of the modern farm cow become concentrated in their milk. These substances, ingested by or injected into the cow, include hormones like IGF (insulin-like growth factor), rBGH (bovine growth hormone), oestrone sulfate, antibiotics, pollutants such as PCBs and dioxin, and a disturbingly long list of many other chemicals, many of which are potential carcinogens or cancer promoters.

Furthermore, commercial production of milk has some questionable practices. For example, the cows may be milked even while they are pregnant, during which their hormone levels are much higher than normal. These hormones are concentrated in milk, and then we drink them. Milk is intended to make a baby grow. Would it be surprising to find that it encourages cancer to grow, too?

On the other hand, human population studies have not confirmed a clear increase in cancer among dairy consumers. Some do report an increased risk, but others show a reduced risk. Also, certain ethnic groups with a traditionally high dairy intake, such as the Maasai, do not seem to have a high cancer rate. Presumably they have favourable genetics which harmonize with their lifestyle[24], and they are drinking raw organic milk, which is quite different to milk from the supermarket.

Soy

Soy is another controversial item. Some will advocate soy as an anticancer food because it contains genistein which can block oestrogen, and is consumed in eastern countries where cancer rates are generally lower.

Those against soy point out that it also has some pro-oestrogenic activity. It contains aluminium, various toxins, and phytic acid which can reduce absorption of calcium and magnesium. It is often genetically modified which usually means that is exposed to high levels of pesticides and herbicides.

Be cautious with dairy and soy. Fermented soy products like soy sauce, miso and tempeh are considered to be okay. Organic unprocessed milk from a non-pregnant grass-fed cow is probably healthy, provided it is from an individual cow or small herd known to be disease free. If you are in a high risk group for cancer, you might consider eliminating dairy and soy altogether, or having them in small amounts, or infrequently. If your cancer risk is not high, you need not be as strict, but don't make them a major part of your diet. Do more reading and make up your own mind. It should be pointed out that these are major industries that protect their own interests, market their products extensively, and have exerted considerable influence on health education and policy.

Summary

Alcohol and red meat increase cancer risk by a small amount, if consumed frequently. Occasional use probably makes little difference, although avoiding processed red meat is a good idea. Sugar and carbohydrates such as refined white flour are more of a concern, carrying a cancer risk via glycaemic load, insulin and IGF. They also lead to obesity which is definitely a major cancer risk factor. There's not much point in giving up hot dogs, or sugar in your coffee, while ignoring the fact that you are overweight. The weight is a bigger danger.

Key Points

- Cancer risk is increased by regular daily consumption of alcohol or red meat.
- The absolute risk is increased by 1% for every alcoholic drink per day, and by 1% for every serve of processed meat per day.
- Processed meat such as bacon, salami, sausage, and hot dogs, should be minimized.
- Unprocessed meat also poses a risk which will likely be reduced by choosing organic meat from grass-fed cows.
- Avoid or minimize added sugar, soft drinks (sodas), sweets (candy), refined white flour (white bread, pastry, biscuits, cakes) and excessive carbohydrates in general.
- The occasional consumption of any of the above will not hurt you.
- Being overweight is a significant cancer risk.

16. HOW TO EAT

Let's consider some practical issues in using nutrition to achieve a cancer-resistant environment in your body. We have already looked at which food to choose, and in each section there are points on preparation. This section complements those points. The focus is on preventing cancer, but of course the general health benefits will be much broader.

Cooking Meat

Cooking meat can produce HCAs (heterocyclic amines) and PAHs (polycyclic aromatic hydrocarbons). These are carcinogenic in animals but this has not been proven in humans. Even so, it would be wise to minimize exposure to them.

The HCAs are produced when meat is cooked at high temperatures, and the PAHs are formed when meat juices drip onto coals, creating fumes that re-enter the food. The main culprit is the barbeque, especially when charring occurs, but high temperatures from frying and broiling will do it too. Stewing, boiling and steaming produce negligible amounts of these toxins because the temperature is much lower. Roasting can produce them because of the long cooking time.

HCAs come only from muscle meats. Other proteins like eggs, cheese or organ meats are okay. Vegetables don't form HCAs either.

Marinades reduce production of HCAs significantly[1]. Beer, wine, lemon or lime can be used, and the effect is even better with herbs and spices such as oregano, rosemary, garlic, ginger, thyme or chilli. Even cherries were shown to lower HCAs significantly. For this effect, the meat does not need to be marinated for hours. Marinades are effective even if applied just before cooking. Also,

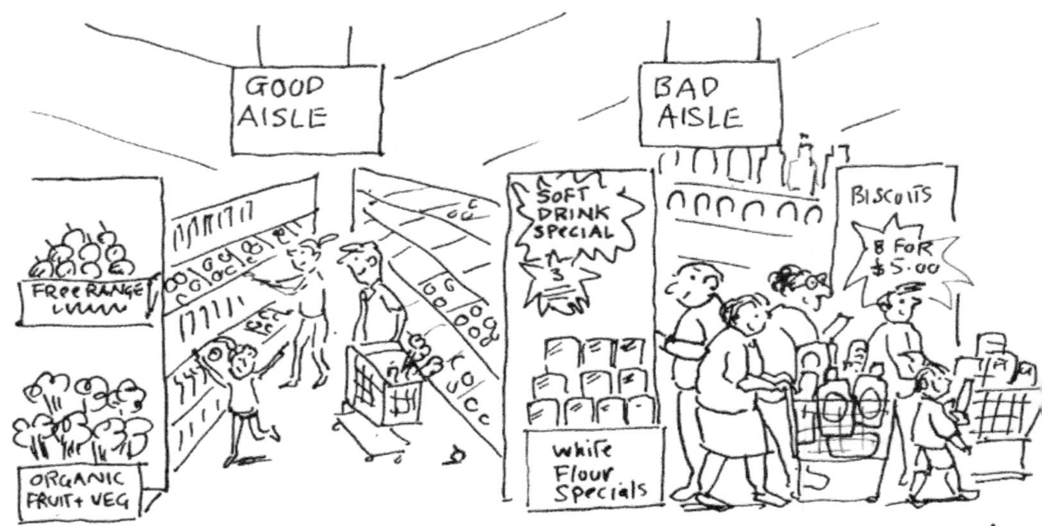

Shop at the periphery of the supermarket to avoid processed food.

crucifer vegetables (such as broccoli) help to detoxify any HCAs that are ingested.

Microwaves and Non-stick Pans

There have been concerns that microwave cooking causes cancer and destroys nutrients, including the ones capable of blocking cancer. However, the research frequently quoted was never published, and the authors and institutions have vanished[2]. There is no firm evidence against microwaves, and there is evidence to show that nutrients are actually quite well preserved compared to other cooking methods[3-5].

The microwave will destroy nutrients if used with higher or prolonged temperatures, or if water is added. Any cooking method using water will result in nutrients moving out of the food and into the water, where they evaporate or are poured away. Do not allow plastic wrap to contact the food and don't use plastic containers that are not microwave approved. These things can certainly produce toxins in the microwave.

Non-stick pans can release toxins. This will happen if the temperature is too high or if the surface is damaged. Avoid using the maximum temperature, and don't leave an empty pan on the heat. Throw the pan away if it is old or the surface is worn or damaged.

Raw versus Cooked

This is a much discussed subject. The proponents of raw food say that cooking destroys nutrients, and also destroys plant enzymes that help to digest the food. Certainly, most fruits and many vegetables can be eaten raw. Others are rather difficult to eat raw, such as pumpkin, sweet potato, onions, beans, lentils, rice, quinoa, etc. Some raw foods are potentially unhealthy, such as mushrooms. Herbs and spices are most easily incorporated in a cooked meal. Would you take a turmeric, pepper and olive oil mixture cold? Tomatoes provide the best protection from cancer when in a cooked form, and tea must be infused into hot water.

Carrots, for example, must be chewed well if raw. Plant cells have a wall of cellulose which needs to be broken to release nutrients for absorption. If not, the nutrients will be carried out with the bowel waste. The cell wall is softened by cooking and much less chewing is required. Most people have an adequate supply of digestive enzymes from the pancreas gland, so enzymes contained within the plant itself (e.g. plant amylase) are not so important, and may not survive passage through the stomach anyway.

Vegetables should be cooked only lightly. Steaming for five minutes or so is an excellent method, softening the food but retaining colour, flavour and nutrients. Brief scalding in hot water works well too, as opposed to prolonged boiling which loses more food value than almost any other cooking method. Roasting or grilling vegetables applies more heat than steaming, but the nutrient loss won't be excessive and the flavours are well preserved. Stir frying (sautéing) is okay because it is quick, but lengthy high-temperature frying will destroy many nutrients.

The aim is to fill your plate with as many anticancer foods as possible. Have them either cooked or raw depending on what is known about that particular food. Many will be beneficial eaten either way, and the cooking method may depend on the meal and what suits you. Don't make too much fuss, and why not cover all bases? If there is any uncertainty, cook in a variety of ways and eat plenty of raw food as well.

Juicing

Juicing is a great way to gain a large quantity and variety of phytochemicals. It allows you to add a wider range of vegetables, and to introduce some that you would not otherwise eat.

For those actively fighting an illness, supranutritional doses can be achieved - i.e. more than you ordinarily need. There are some potential problems with this. Firstly, you need to introduce juicing gradually otherwise it may make you feel unwell. Secondly, everything in the plant is concentrated, both the good and the bad. That includes residues of pesticides and fertilizers. So, if you are drinking serious quantities of juice, organically grown produce is advised. Also, if you are making such an effort, make sure that the produce is of high quality in other aspects. Where was it grown? How old is it? How was it transported? Organic just means no artificial chemicals. It does not guarantee nutritional quality. Organic has many definitions. Does the product comply with organic standards?

We are talking here about making your own juice, as opposed to commercial juice which has been processed and will often lack any worthwhile nutrition. Try making your own apple juice and then ask why the commercial product looks so different. It looks clear because the phytochemicals have been filtered out, otherwise they oxidize and go brown, leaving a haze or sediment, which the manufacturers don't like.

What about orange juice? Whole oranges are preferable to juice. Fruit juice has very high sugar content, with one big glass having the juice of about four oranges, and nearly as much sugar (24g) as fizzy soft drinks (30g). Most juices lack fibre, although some will be present if the pulp is added back. Many major commercial brands are processed to provide a uniform flavour, whatever the season. This is done by keeping it in large vats for several months, mixing new with old, deoxygenating it to prevent degradation, and then artificially adding back flavour. The flavouring is not mentioned on the label if it is derived from orange essences or oil.

The sugar load is a concern with juicing, as opposed to eating the whole fruit or vegetable. For one thing, juice may simply contain too much sugar, particularly if much fruit is used. That is why vegetables are advocated for juicing, with just a small amount of fruit to add flavour. In addition, un-juiced whole food simply can't be consumed as fast, and contains more fibre, both of which result in delayed absorption and a more gradual uptake of sugar, avoiding the spikes in blood sugar and insulin levels which can occur with juice alone.

The juice should be consumed soon after being made, otherwise the nutrients degrade (oxidize), but it can be kept in an airtight container in the fridge for 24 hours.

There are two main types of juicer. The most common is the high speed blending type which has the advantage of being very fast and retaining the fibre. However, it is possible that the high speed may destroy some nutrients. Some people prefer a slow speed "masticating" type. This mimics a human chew, but does it much better. The phytochemicals will be very well preserved, but the fibre is lost, which is no problem as long as you get fibre from the rest of your diet. However, these juicers can be tedious to use because the fruit and vegetables need to be chopped into small pieces that are fed in individually, and the juice is produced quite slowly.

Many of the foods covered in this book do not lend themselves to juicing. Consider apples, carrots, celery, and pineapple for juicing if you use a masticating type of juicer. They all have anticancer properties. Foods like spinach, parsley, ginger, and certain berries will be better in the high speed type of juicer because they make more of a pulp than actual juice. There are plenty of juicing and smoothie recipes available. Just try a few combinations in whatever juicer you have, aiming to use the best foods against cancer. It is not necessary to insist on perfection. You are more likely to participate if your juice is not too laborious to produce and tastes alright.

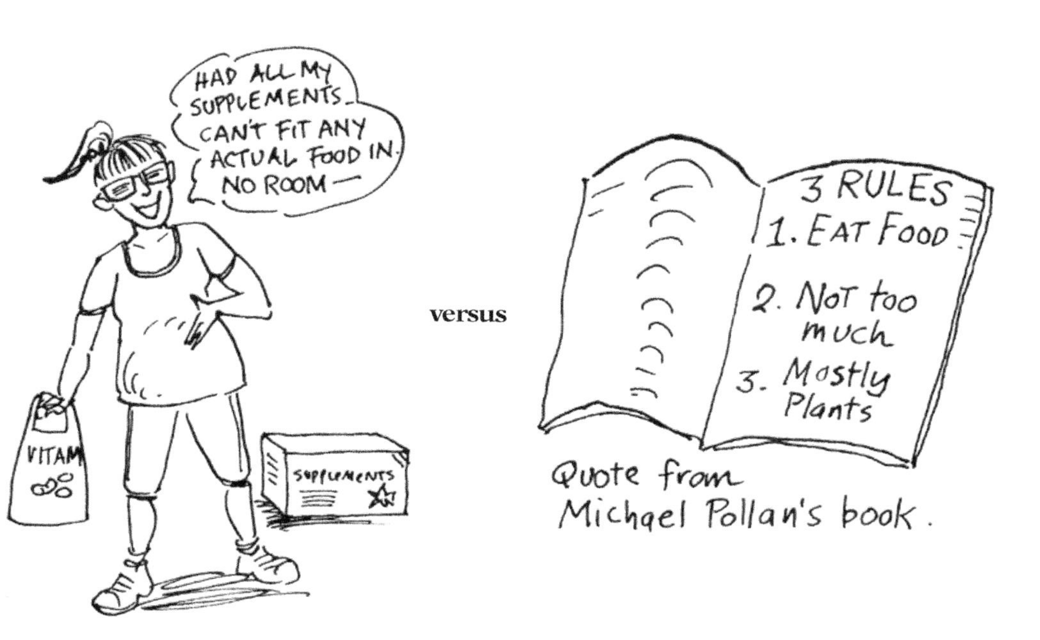

Breakfast and Snack Options

I have not included recipes in this book, but have provided some useful sources in the appendix. However, I will make some specific suggestions with regard to breakfast and snacks between meals, because these mealtimes can be particularly unhealthy in western countries.

Unfortunately, a western-culture breakfast tends to be carbohydrate-based, such as refined white-flour bread or boxed cereals which are so processed that vitamins need to be added back in. Remember, vitamins in supplement form don't reduce cancer risk. They need to be in whole food. Breakfast cereals are often excessively sweetened. They are consumed with large volumes of milk which has also been depleted of food value, and may itself increase cancer risk. Breakfast often includes commercial fruit juice which is another big sugar load. All this sugar and the insulin that follows, can't be good. The problem is that many people in western culture can't imagine anything else for breakfast. How did it get this way? The answer is that it is quick, convenient and aggressively marketed. Processed food is more profitable. Not only is this popular breakfast not very good for you, but you are missing the opportunity to have some cancer-fighting food.

If you need some ideas, consider-

- Scrambled eggs with tomato and herbs
- Oats with yoghurt and dried fruit
- Shredded coconut, ground flax seeds, Brazil nuts, berries and almond milk
- Steamed greens and quinoa
- Omelette with mushrooms and spinach

These don't exclusively feature food types from the anticancer list, but at least one of the components you will recognize as such, and with some thought you can do more. For example, you could use turmeric, pepper and olive oil with the eggs. Make a habit of having an orange or apple. You can drink green tea while you are preparing breakfast (catechins are absorbed well on an empty stomach). Allow enough time in the morning. This might mean waking earlier to avoid a stressful rush. Maybe someone else in the house wants to join in and help out if it is a cooked breakfast.

Plan what snacks you will have between meals, too. As with breakfast, a bad snack choice puts you a step back, while a good choice puts you a step forward, which adds up to being two steps ahead. Every time you eat something unhelpful, it has taken the place of something beneficial. Small habits will amount to a big difference over a long period of time.

Consider having a ready supply of fruit and vegetables in the house that require no preparation and can be taken with you to work. Otherwise, you will buy and eat something unhelpful or detrimental instead. Other anticancer snack examples include sardines, yoghurt with ground flax seeds, nuts (Brazil nuts, walnuts, almonds, pistachios) or nut butter on pieces of apple or celery.

Eating Attitudes and New Behaviours

Are you conscious of what you eat? What is actually in it? Where did it come from? How much has it been interfered with (processed)? What is in it that is good for me? This is eating consciously. Intuition is when you seem to know something without necessarily having been handed the information directly. "Intuitive eating" involves listening to your body and developing a sense of what it is really crying out for. Old habits might push you towards a sweet snack, but maybe your body is just asking for a glass of water.

Be patient with yourself. Some things can be changed instantly, while others take gradual adjustment or may never work for you. Don't consider yourself to be on a diet. You are just adopting a new way of "seeing" food.

Developing a healthy lifestyle does require a decision and then discipline to follow through and maintain it, but don't be so strict that you are always thinking about it. Don't worry about food so much that you feel stressed. That would be counterproductive because stress weakens your immune system.

If you are giving up junk food and fizzy drinks and trying to lose weight, you will experience cravings. Sometimes eating has become a habit that we obey without actually being hungry. Or it can be a way of dealing with emotions, even though you might not be in genuine physical need of food. You may need to get in touch with yourself in order to involve your conscious mind in your behaviours. As you over-ride your subconscious, you are re-programming it, and soon it will come on side. This is letting the captain decide on the direction of the ship, instead of the unruly crew.

A degree of flexibility is appropriate. If you deprive yourself completely, the cravings may become unbearable, eventually overwhelming you and leaving a feeling of guilt. You can do without that! So have a few treats, but steer yourself to healthier ones. Soon you will actually lose a taste for rubbish. You will look at the food in your hand and realize that you are not even enjoying it the way you used to. Your body is telling you what it really needs instead. Then when you do indulge through choice, you are less likely to overdo it, compared to when you have been fighting so hard that when the dam wall breaks, it does so in a major way. If you do binge, forgive yourself; remind yourself of the healthy food which you enjoy and aim to go that way next time.

Recognize when you are hungry and when you have had enough. When your stomach is full, stop eating (or preferably before that point). If you eat too fast, you may miss the signal and then overeat.

Periodic fasting has proven health benefits[6,7]. This can be as an intermittent fast in which you miss two consecutive meals - e.g. have your evening meal, and then nothing till the evening meal the next day. This will give you a better awareness of what genuine hunger feels like, and it helps you to see food as nourishment rather than just as a routine. Another idea is to specifically restrict your carbohydrate intake for two days every week. These methods will help you lose weight if you need to, but may backfire if you gorge yourself the rest of the time. If you have decided to eat less meat, try having two or three days a week without it.

Avoid rushing meals while travelling to work or standing in front of the fridge. Instead, focus for a minute on the healthy nourishment you are bringing to yourself. Savour the texture and flavour of your food. Imagine all those phytochemicals mixing together, destined to work in synergy against cancer as they move into your body. Mealtimes can be an opportunity for some peace, as we take a relaxing, healing break from our hectic world.

BOX: FOOD CONTAMINANTS – AVOID OR REMOVE

The main advantage of organically-produced food is the absence of harmful chemicals. If you are not using organic plants, be aware that certain fruits and vegetables are known to be more contaminated than others.

According to the Environmental Working Group[8], the "dirty dozen" for 2014 are:

- Apples
- Strawberries
- Grapes
- Celery
- Peaches
- Spinach
- Sweet bell peppers
- Nectarines
- Cucumbers
- Cherry tomatoes
- Snap peas
- Potatoes

The "Clean Fifteen" for 2014 (least likely to hold pesticide residues) are:

- Avocados
- Sweet corn
- Pineapples
- Cabbage
- Peas
- Onions
- Asparagus
- Mangoes
- Pawpaws
- Kiwifruit
- Eggplant

- Grapefruit
- Cantaloupe
- Cauliflower
- Sweet potatoes

Broccoli and cauliflower are quite clean, and anything that is peeled (oranges, bananas, avocado) will be fairly safe. However, chemicals can't be completely removed by washing, and there will still be some on the inside of the plant from absorption during its growth.

Certain crops are nearly always heavily treated by the farmer to counter specific agricultural problems, but there will be variation between geographical locations and farmers.

All fruits and vegetables should be washed. Those least contaminated can be quickly rinsed. The worst ones can be cleaned more thoroughly. If they are smooth (e.g. apples, cucumbers), a brisk wash with tap water and a firm dry with a cloth will suffice. If the shape is irregular (e.g. grapes, strawberries), you can use a very small amount of detergent, then rinse until the water is clear. A step further would be to buy a commercial cleaner or make your own with salt or vinegar. However, if you are that concerned, just buy organic for the produce that is known to be most contaminated or difficult to clean well.

In addition, you can learn the best way to reduce ingestion of contaminants from the specific food that you eat the most. For example, apples (the worst on the list) can be managed by not eating the area around the stalk where residues accumulate, but don't remove the peel because it is the best part.

Be aware that there are well described standards required for the label of organic to be used, but some sellers may apply the standards more loosely than others, so you need to be discerning. Also, produce grown locally, in good soil, and harvested and delivered in season may be more nutritious than organic produce if it is picked unripe, transported long distances, or stored for lengthy periods.

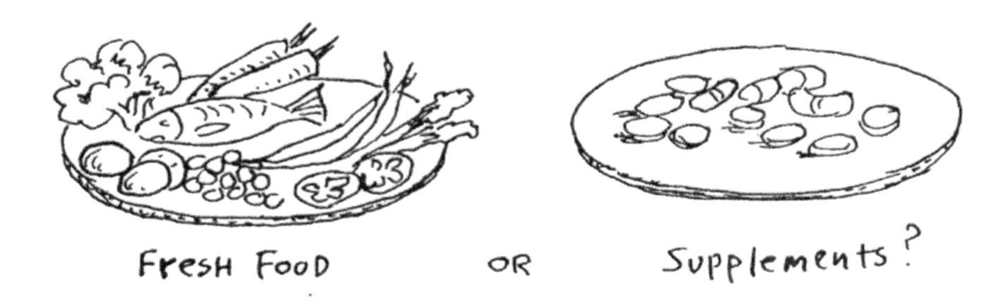

BOX: SYNERGY VERSUS SUPPLEMENTS

Synergy refers to two or more elements working together to produce an effect greater than the sum of their individual effects.

Synergism can result in increased effectiveness of compounds by ten times or more. It may be by direct chemical interaction but it can also be via improved absorption, by working at different points in the cancer sequence (promotion or progression), or by complementary mechanisms (one blocks cancer blood vessel growth and another is an immune booster).

This provides a way in which a clinical effect can be achieved despite apparently poor blood levels.

For example, the effects of curcumin are dose-dependent, meaning that the higher the levels, the greater the end effect. Because it is difficult to achieve high blood levels, we can take advantage of synergy to get the same result with lower levels. Curcumin is synergistic with resveratrol in grapes, EGCG in green tea, and garcinol in mangosteen (against pancreatic cancer cells). PE-ITC from sulforaphane in broccoli is synergistic with curcumin in causing apoptosis (cell death) in prostate cancer cells. Piperine from black pepper improves the absorption of curcumin.

Many synergisms between phytochemicals acting against cancer have been recognized, and it is likely that there are many yet to be identified. This highlights the importance of consuming a wide variety of plants in natural combinations. The term "whole foods" means that the complete plant source is available, rather than purified components. Synergism is able to occur between the chemicals within each whole food, and with those in other whole plant foods consumed in the same meal (or even at other times, if they linger for a while).

On the other hand, potential synergy may be lost if purified "active ingredients" have been separated from other substances in food. This is one reason why supplements may not have the effectiveness of the whole natural source. Certainly this has been shown repeatedly for garlic supplements as opposed to actual whole garlic. In fact, some multivitamin preparations contain substances that actually work against each other.

Supplementation is often used to achieve doses that cannot be achieved through normal eating. This sounds good, but can be detrimental. For example, carrots provide vitamin A and carotenes which both have anticancer effects. However, vitamin A supplements are able to result in much higher blood levels than what can be achieved with food, and these high levels are actually toxic. Also, beta-carotene supplements were shown to increase lung cancer risk, in contrast to whole food sources. Fibre taken as a supplement may do more harm than good.

Other issues with supplements are reliability of dosage and quality control, degradation during storage and transport, and expense.

There are some exceptions where supplements are expected to be favourable. Firstly, some extracts have been demonstrated as helpful in clinical settings – e.g. mushroom extracts and their purified beta-glucans. Secondly, certain elements have become deficient in our diets, and supplementing these will be beneficial because they have a critical role in healthy cell function (e.g. selenium, magnesium, iodine).

In "The China Study"[9], Colin Campbell asks us to imagine a mouthful of "sautéed spinach with ginger and whole grain ravioli shells stuffed with butternut squash and spices, topped with a walnut sauce". He describes how, with chewing and digestion, this becomes a complex mixture of thousands of food chemicals interacting with each other in ways beyond what we will ever fully understand. How could we expect to use a handful of encapsulated nutrients or active ingredients to imitate this?

Key Points

- Charring meat at high temperatures in a frying pan or on a barbeque produces carcinogenic toxins. These can be negated by marinating with beer, wine, lemon, lime or spices.
- Microwave cooking does not destroy or waste nutrients unless too much water is used.
- Microwaves may generate toxins from plastic wrap or incorrect cookware.
- Non-stick pans release toxins if used at maximum temperature or if the surface is worn or damaged.
- In most cases, it is not important whether plants are eaten raw or cooked, but light cooking preserves nutrients well. Boiling is the worst method.
- Juicing is an effective way of achieving a high dose of plant nutrients. Organic or thoroughly washed plants should be used. Use less fruit than vegetables to avoid excessive sugar. Commercial juices provide negligible anticancer nutrition.
- Replace a breakfast of bread, cereal and milk with foods like eggs, yoghurt, fruit, nuts and seeds.
- Allow time to introduce the necessary changes to your lifestyle. Construct a plan and be disciplined, but remain flexible and don't get stressed over it. Be conscious of what you eat.
- Supplements are generally less effective against cancer than whole foods which contain a multitude of substances acting in synergy.

17. THE "FOOD IS MEDICINE" ACTION PLAN

Steps to Take

Now is your chance to do something!

To help you convert this knowledge into action, I have made some suggestions. If you are already on the right track, that is great. But if you want to change, these ideas might help. The main thing is that you actually start somewhere, even with something small. Persist with the first step, then gradually introduce new habits.

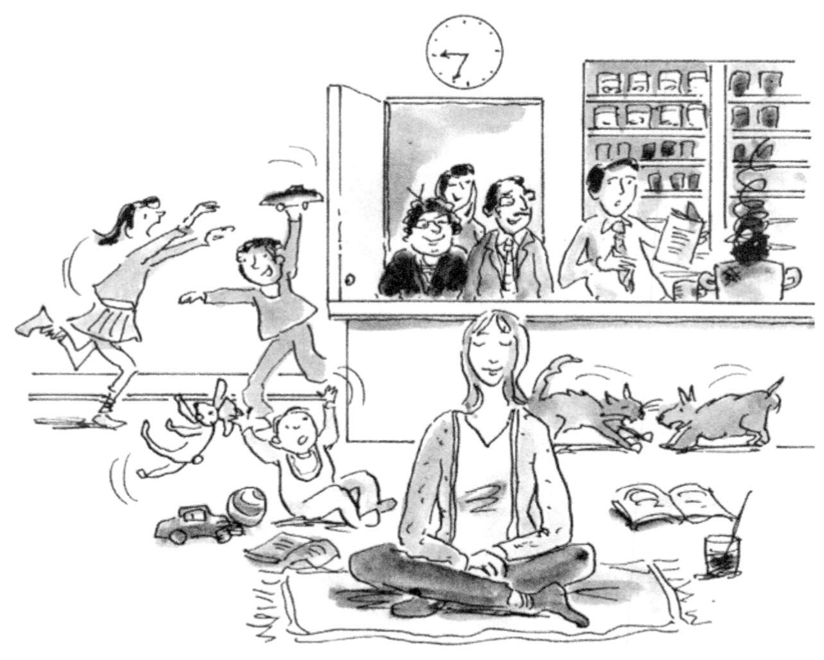

It should be enjoyable and sustainable, rather than a painful chore.

Here is a plan of action. Tackle one point at a time, in whatever order appeals to you.

1. Anticancer food with every meal
2. More veges, less meat, less carbs
3. Snack against cancer
4. Overhaul your breakfast
5. Drink green tea
6. Stock up with good stuff
7. Give up the bad
8. Supplement with selenium and vitamin D
9. Find a healthy restaurant
10. Don't go it alone

Cancer is a chronic illness, meaning that it takes years to form, and usually is quite slow to progress. You have time to act. Make the changes one by one if you like, but make them for good. A new habit takes three weeks to form, and after that, it is easier to maintain. Write down what you want to do, and make goals with timeframes. Be aware of what you are buying, and what you are putting on the table. What you see on your plate is a constant reminder of your progress. Soon enough you will have achieved your goals. You will also be exercising your body and learning mindfulness as part of your overall plan. Don't demand too much, or overload yourself with tasks. Slow and steady will win this race.

Let's look at some details.

1. Have at least one anticancer food with every meal, and add new items to your diet.

   What vegetables and fruit do you already like? They nearly all have some anticancer properties, but some are better than others. Are you already eating some of the most effective foods? If so, increase the quantity of these and start adding some of the ones that you don't usually eat. For example, let's consider a popular salad consisting of carrots, tomatoes, celery and cucumber. Tomatoes and carrots are definitely on our list. Even celery and cucumber may have some anticancer value, although they are not key players. Perhaps you could add some spring onions, parsley, baby spinach, green beans, snow peas, radishes, sprouts, broccoli, cabbage or avocado. All these have anticancer phytochemicals.

Make a list of the anticancer foods that you want to add to your diet, and ask which meals you can incorporate them into. Perhaps try a new one each week. Develop a taste for foods like broccoli and turmeric, and make them regulars in your kitchen. Almost every meal can include onion and garlic. Try new things when you are energetic and motivated, but have some easy "default" meals that you can fall back on at other times.

2. Change food proportions

Eat less meat and starchy vegetables like potato. Have more of other vegetables (these should fill at least half the plate), and have a greater quantity and variety of them. If this is very different to what you are used to, just do it gradually; perhaps start with two meals per week.

3. Snacks

Cancer-fighting foods make great snacks - e.g. fruit, vegetables, nuts, yoghurt, and sardines. You can make a huge salad of the items mentioned above in Point #1, and keep it in a container in the fridge to have whenever you like. Don't use commercial salad dressing; instead, add a little olive oil, vinegar or spices.

4. Breakfast may need to be completely overhauled

This particularly applies if you are a cereal and milk, or toast and juice, person. Look at the ideas in Chapter 16 "How to Eat". Make breakfast enough of a priority that you take the time to prepare it. This is definitely worth the effort.

5. Drink green tea

Green tea can become your choice whenever you are offered a beverage. It won't take long before you prefer it. Try it when you get up in the morning; it is well absorbed on an empty stomach.

6. Stock up

If you don't have beneficial foods in the house, you will end up eating something else. If you live in a western culture, this will typically be something that simply fills your stomach, such as refined carbohydrates (e.g. bread, pasta). Why have those things when they will probably increase cancer risk, while missing out on a dose of preventive medicine? Instead, buy the right stuff and always have plenty of it. Consider having vegetables delivered, perhaps once per week to supplement your regular shopping.

7. Give up

Give up fizzy soft drinks (sodas) and flavoured milk drinks. Minimize white bread, cakes, sweet biscuits and sugary snacks. If you drink alcohol every day, cut back. Quit hot dogs altogether. Minimize bacon, salami and other processed red meat. It won't really hurt to have these things occasionally, but after a while you may lose your desire for them.

8. Supplements – selenium, vitamin D and others

As a principle, whole foods are preferred, but some supplements are worth considering. You have to be selective here, because there are so many supplements, exhaustively recommended and promoted at every turn. Consider taking selenium and magnesium. Vitamin D should be supplemented if your levels are low on testing, and are not easily corrected by sunshine in your particular case. Ask your doctor to test your thyroid function and urine iodine levels. If necessary, boost your iodine intake with seaweed, kelp tablets, or iodine drops. If you are battling cancer, or in a high risk group, think about mushroom extracts and resveratrol as well.

9. Find a restaurant near you with a menu that meets our criteria.

We all like to go out or order take-away (take-out) meals occasionally. With practice, you will be able to choose appropriate meals or even ask the chef to modify a meal. However, not every meal has to be perfectly healthy, so don't be too fussy, particularly if you are with company.

10. Don't go it alone.

Most of the world may be eating rubbish. This can make you feel like you are the only one on this path. We want it to be easy for you to get your "medicine". For example, someone else in the house may be able to do some juicing or make you a nutritious smoothie. Chopping things up and getting all the ingredients together may be too much of a chore, especially if you aren't feeling well. Perhaps a friend will get enthusiastic about growing broccoli sprouts for you, or you could experiment with sauerkraut together.

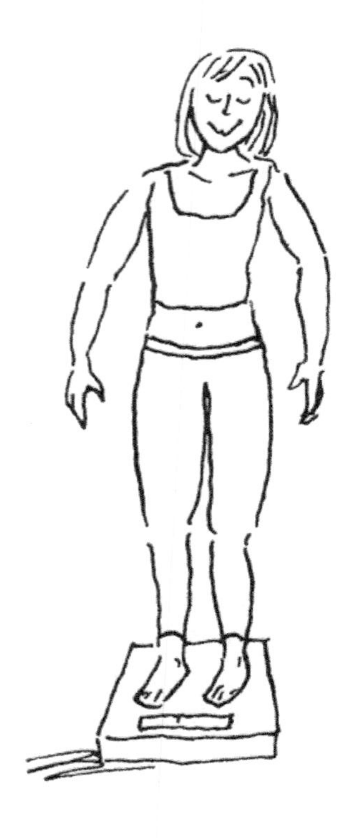

Encourage your husband, wife, or partner to get on board. It is complicated to have separate meals, and making changes can be hard enough without resistance at home. Find at least one other person on the same journey for mutual encouragement, to share the adventure of discovering the anticancer lifestyle, and to keep each other accountable. If you are a cancer patient, your doctor or nurse might be able to match you up with someone with a similar background and interests. There are online forums and discussion groups, too. Place a motivational picture or quote in your house or workplace. Not only does it benefit you, but when people ask about it, you can explain your new knowledge against cancer, and your mission. You will need to give them a progress report next time!

Part of a Bigger Plan

"Food is Medicine" is the foundational lifestyle factor that can be used against cancer, but it does not stand alone. It should be applied in conjunction with other key strategies.

Exercise (and sunshine)

These reduce cancer risk and are part of the plan.

1. Exercise three hours per week. It needn't be onerous, especially if you can build it into your routine. Try walking part of the

way to work by parking further away, or walking to the next bus stop. Walk to school with the kids, or walk the dog. Ride your bike to hire a movie or post a letter. Join in team sport one evening a week and enjoy the social element. Perhaps you are physically active during a normal day anyway. It all counts.

2. Prolonged sessions of strenuous exercise are unnecessary, and can even be harmful in the long term (proinflammatory).
3. Get your vitamin D level checked, and aim to be well above the recommended lower limit. Vitamin D protects against cancer. If your level isn't good enough, get more sunshine. Start with just 10 minutes exposure (or less if it makes you go pink), three times a week. Otherwise, take a supplement (2000 IU per day), and recheck the level after 3 months.

Be peaceful and mindful

Your mind is connected to your body.

1. Keep things in perspective.
2. Live in the moment.
3. Plan for the future and do what you can, then stop worrying.
4. Value relationships and experiences most highly. "The best things in life are... not things"
5. Forgive everyone (deep bitterness or subconscious resentments will affect your physical health, too).
6. Enlarge the spiritual dimension of your life.
7. Learn "mindfulness" and meditation (can be short and simple).

So here we have:

1. Nutrition - (Food is medicine)
2. Exercise and sunshine
3. Your mind

Be active instead of passive. Participate in your own health, knowing that you are on a path of prevention or recovery. Understand what is happening in your body, and feed it what it needs. Be a friend to your stomach and your immune system. Sense a new balanced internal state and enjoy it.

Part Two:
A BIT MORE SCIENCE

18. CANCER CONCEPTS – HOW IT WORKS AND HOW TO STOP IT

Angiogenesis

Angiogenesis refers to the formation of new blood vessels. It is one of the steps required for cancer growth.

Initially, a cancer cell can take its nutrients directly from the surrounding tissues. However, as cancer cells divide and reproduce themselves, they form a mass that now needs blood vessels to bring nutrients into it. Tumours can grow up to about half a millimetre in size without any blood vessels of their own, but once they get any bigger, they can't survive without them.

Cells are able to secrete certain chemical factors that stimulate the growth of new blood vessels. This is angiogenesis. It is a complex multistep process normally tightly controlled, and mainly turned on during normal growth and healing. If angiogenesis in a cancer can be blocked, it will starve and die.

In autopsy studies of people who have died from other (not cancer) causes, it is very common to find microscopic spots of malignant cells in tissues like the breast, the thyroid or the prostate, but these cancer cells have never progressed or caused any harm. It has been suggested that they did not progress because there was no angiogenesis.

Angiogenesis has become a target for cancer treatments. For example, a drug called Avastin works well against blood vessels in certain types of tumours, and it can increase survival times of patients. Similarly, there are factors in food that also block angiogenesis. Resveratrol from grapes, ellagic acid from berries, sulforaphane from broccoli, catechins from green tea, and curcumin in turmeric are all effective. In at least some of these, the effect is synergistic.

A study from Harvard of 79,000 men showed that two or three servings of cooked tomatoes per week reduced the risk of prostate cancer by more than 40%[1]. Tomatoes contain lycopene which is anti-angiogenic. In the men who did develop prostate cancer, the tumours were found to have less blood vessels feeding them than expected.

Sulforaphane in broccoli reduces the formation of new capillaries in lab experiments by interfering with vascular endothelial growth factor (VEGF). When a cell is not getting enough oxygen, hypoxia factors are produced which go to the cell nucleus and induce transcription of the VEGF gene. This leads to production of VEGF protein which is then released from the cell. It binds to the surface of nearby blood vessel cells, stimulating them to grow and feed the cancer. As the cancer grows, it continues to bring new blood vessels with it by this process. Sulforaphane has been shown to downregulate (block) transcription of the VEGF gene, as well as blocking the VEGF receptor itself and the hypoxia factors.

The concept is beautifully explained on an Internet site called TED.com by William Li[2,3]. The whole point of his lecture was that anti-angiogenic compounds occur naturally in foods. What amazed me was that at the end of his presentation, the question the moderator asked him was about the development of drugs that can do this, which disregarded his whole point about the potential of food.

Not all cancers rely on VEGF, and there are other ways in which cancers are able to stimulate angiogenesis, so blocking VEGF is not a magic cure. Nutrition provides many phytochemicals with multiple modes of action against cancer. This is just one way the correct food might help.

Apoptosis

The term "apoptosis" comes from an ancient Greek word applied to the process of leaves dropping off a tree. Like a dead or damaged leaf dropping off, an unhealthy cell is removed by apoptosis, also described as programmed cell suicide.

In fact, millions of damaged or unneeded cells disappear from the average person's body in this way, every day. Having the appropriate number of cells depends on the balance between cell proliferation

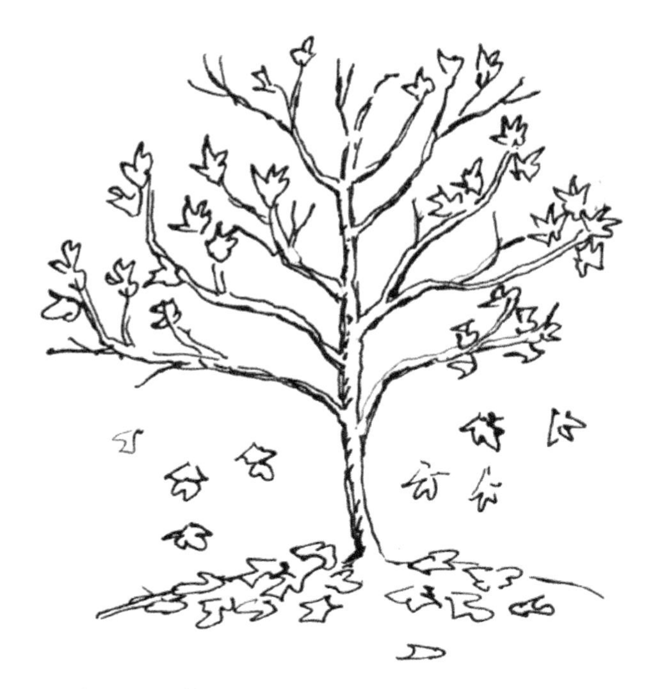

(production of new cells) and apoptosis. Cancers usually have both increased proliferation and decreased apoptosis, and cancer treatments are aimed at turning these around.

The cancer drug, Gleevec, works by triggering apoptosis (by inhibiting tyrosine kinase). Most anticancer foods exert their effects, at least in part, via apoptosis, and are able to do so via several different pathways. Normal cells are not affected.

For example, DADS from garlic and sulforaphane from broccoli activate p53. This is a tumour suppressor gene that causes cell cycle arrest (the cell becomes frozen part way through the process of dividing). At this point, attempts to repair the cancer cell DNA are made, but if unsuccessful, the cell is driven to self destruct (apoptosis).

Many cancers end up with a mutation of the p53 gene in their cells, leading to a mutated p53 protein that actually blocks apoptosis instead of promoting it. Sulforaphane (in broccoli) is converted to another chemical called phenylethyl-ITC (PE-ITC) which binds to mutant p53, and allows apoptosis to occur.

Plant chemicals also induce apoptosis by other mechanisms, including activation of caspase enzymes which break down internal cell organelles. The disintegrating cell is then consumed by nearby white cells, and that's it. Gone.

Antioxidants

When I first mention in conversation that I am writing about how certain foods work against cancer, a common response is, "Oh yes... antioxidants." Everyone seems to know the word and that we need plenty of them to be healthy. I then stress that there are many other ways in which plants fight cancer. Antioxidants are important but they are not the only factor. In fact, supplements containing specific antioxidants in isolation may even be detrimental.

Antioxidants block oxidation. Why are we worried about "oxidation"? Is it related to oxygen? Isn't oxygen a good thing?

It's interesting to learn that although we use oxygen to generate energy and life, its reactions can also lead to destruction. Think of rust, which is the oxidation of iron. Oxygen is very reactive, and its reactions produce "reactive oxygen species", including "free radicals". These can cause damage to cells and DNA. Oxidative damage to DNA can cause cancer. Our bodies have in-built antioxidant systems to remove these chemicals before they cause damage.

Plants are rich in antioxidants to protect themselves from the by-products of photosynthesis. When we eat plants, the ingested antioxidants aid our internal systems, too.

Perhaps the best known antioxidants in food are vitamin C and beta-carotene, both of which are in a wide variety of fruit and vegetables. Another favourite is ellagic acid in blueberries. These all directly mop up or "scavenge" free radicals. Selenium is a vital component of the glutathione system, one of our key internal antioxidant systems. As mentioned, the genes which control the glutathione system are favourably regulated by plant chemicals such as sulforaphane in broccoli which turns on the gene for glutathione enzymes.

Antioxidant activity is important, but is only one component of the cancer protection offered by plants, which have an abundance of phytochemicals working in many other ways, too.

Genetic Mutations in Cancer Cells

A study of cells in oesophageal cancer in rats looked at the effect of black raspberry extract on "bad genes". The authors write (take a deep breath!):

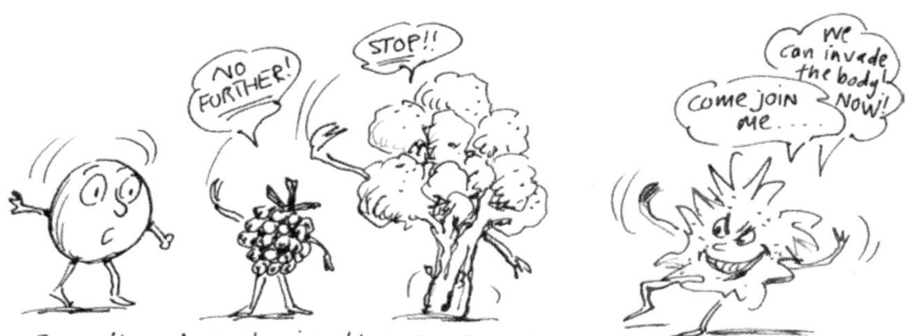

Broccoli and raspberries block the transformation of a happy healthy cell into an ugly angry malignant cell.

"The conversion of a normal cell into a tumorigenic cell is driven by numerous molecular aberrations that arise over time that endow the ultimate cell with resistance to apoptosis, insensitivity to growth-inhibitory signals, limitless replicative potential, sustained angiogenesis, and tissue invasion or metastatic capabilities."[4]

What they are saying is that a normal cell has many fine controls, or "checks and balances" which govern when it should grow or divide. However, these controls are gradually lost in the progression from normal to malignant. The first genetic change may result in the cell losing its ability to inactivate carcinogens (chemicals which cause cancer). The carcinogen may then cause another change in the cell's genetics which allows a slightly abnormal cell to go on living when it should have self-destructed (apoptosis). A further genetic mutation allows it to divide and reproduce, ignoring the body's chemical messengers giving "no grow" signals. Still more mutations block the usual chemistry that should repair errors in the genes. Soon this new clone of cells is reproducing itself, uncontrolled.

Because these cells are abnormal, they have inefficient metabolism which leads to low oxygen levels and increased acidity, making them "sicker" and allowing further genetic damage to occur. Now the cells acquire the ability to move through blood vessel walls and spread through the body because their mutated surface ignores the rules that govern polite cell behaviour. They lose normal adhesion to adjacent cells, become motile and break through cell junctions. Meanwhile more mutations continue to occur. Some of these allow the cell to release chemicals which stimulate blood vessels to grow into the enlarging mass to feed it (angiogenesis). The mutations are not intentional or directed in any way. They are random, but prolific enough for the occasional one to be beneficial to cancer cell survival. Many other mutations contribute to the cell eventually becoming unrecognisable (i.e. poorly differentiated, high grade).

In the black raspberry experiment, the cancer cells were found to have 2,261 dysregulated (changed or out of control) genes. That's not a misprint - over two thousand! That's a lot of bad genes. When they exposed the cells to a broccoli extract, 1323 of those bad genes were normalized. When they applied black raspberries, 462 genes were normalized - not as good as broccoli but still pretty useful. Some of the genes affected were those which controlled apoptosis, cell division, angiogenesis, and inactivation of carcinogens. In the fight against cancer, not all the abnormal genes need to be corrected, but enough to cause those cells to die or stop dividing. The cell has a very complex engine, and damaging just one element can shut the whole thing down.

We have been living with plants on this planet for a long time, but we have been gradually eliminating whole unprocessed fresh plants from our diet. We have focused too much on the basic "building blocks" of protein, carbohydrate, fats and vitamins, while ignoring the importance of the chemistry of phytonutrients in regulating cell growth, genetic stability, and even genetic expression. Our grandparents knew that optimal health required exercise, sunshine and vegetables. We ignored them because we judged them to be from an unscientific age, and now science is proving that they were right all along!

Signalling Pathways

For a cell to perform a particular function or to manufacture something, it will often require a signal or chain of relayed signals. This is referred to as a signalling pathway, and there are many such pathways in a cell. They are initiated by a substance that comes into contact with the cell via the bloodstream, or from the immediate cellular environment. The substance locks onto a receptor on the cell surface, leading to a cascade of chemical reactions within the cell cytoplasm. After a number of steps, a final chemical is released which is able to enter the nucleus where it comes into contact with

Figure: Signalling pathway concept

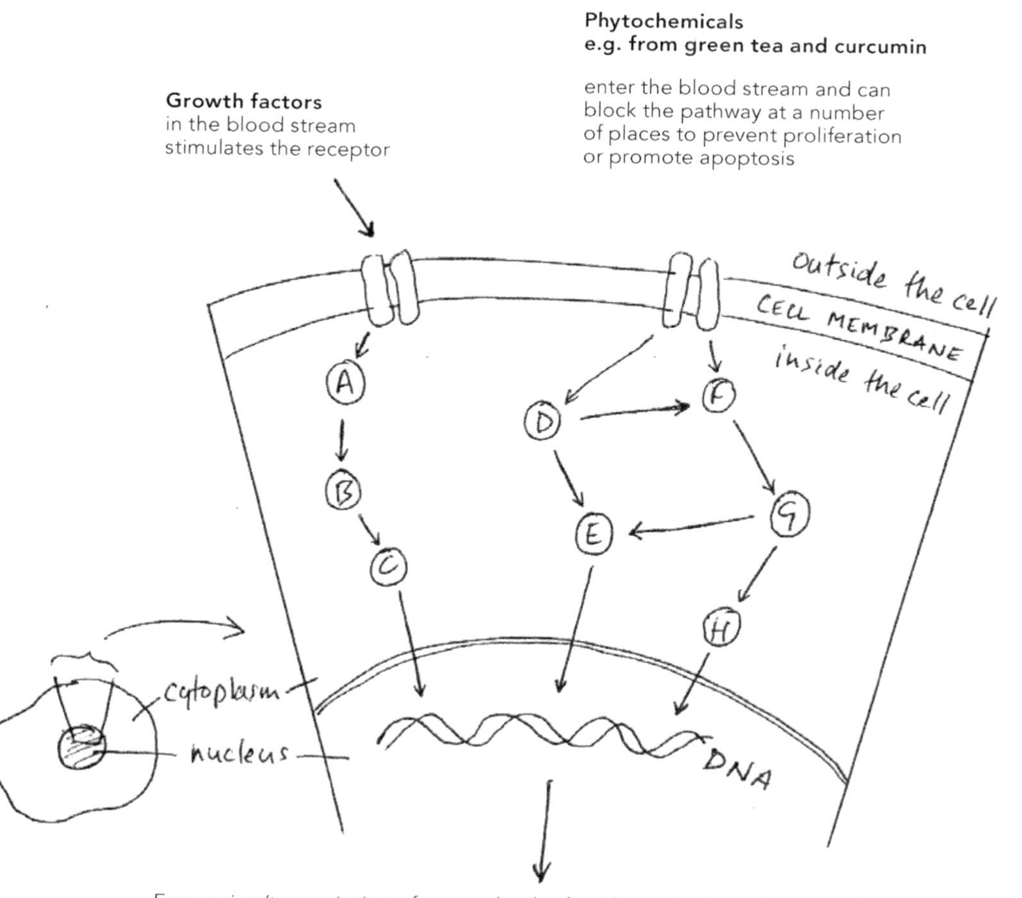

Expression/transcription of a gene by the final factor in the pathway leads to:
cell division/proliferation
apoptosis
angiogenesis
migration/invasion
(depending which particular gene has been turned on or off)

The letters A to H represent various chemicals in the pathway, each of which becomes activated, and in turn activates the next step in the signalling chain, leading to a final factor which enters the nucleus to activate (or deactivate) a gene. Note that there are several interacting pathways. Phytochemicals may be able to block the cascade at several points to prevent cancer initiation or progression. To see some actual examples on the internet, search for images of "signalling pathways."

the cell's DNA (genes). This results in expression of a specific gene, usually leading to production of whatever that particular cell is supposed to do as its normal function in the body.

With respect to cancer growth, expression of genes may lead to cell division, angiogenesis, or other enablements to enhance survival. There is the potential for any of the steps in the sequence to be blocked, to prevent cancer growth. Pharmaceutical companies aim to develop drugs to block these points. The problem is that the malignant cell gets around it by "finding" alternative pathways. Actually, it can't "plan" how to do this. What happens is that the cancer environment is so toxic or the internal function of the cell so deranged, that DNA damage is ongoing. This multitude of random mutations occurring in thousands of cells in the tumour mass eventually leads to one or more of those cells developing the necessary variation in a signalling pathway to bypass the block. The cells which have the new pathway survive and multiply. This becomes the new successful clone. And so the cancer lives on, despite the initial effectiveness of the drug in causing signal blockade. This is one reason why certain cancer treatments may work well for a while, but later fail. In contrast to a drug, which is a single chemical with a specific target, dietary components are immense in their variety of chemical structures. This enables them to act on many different signalling pathways, and at many levels of these pathways, in order to block tumour growth. Green tea is a great example (see p.161).

Food chemicals will not have the immediate potency of drugs, but can be exerting a continuous background effect over many years.

Inflammation

Recently there has been recognition of a causal link between inflammation and the development of cancer[5-9]. Why would this be the case?

Cancer has been described as "the wound that does not heal". Certainly cancers which result in ulceration and an open wound often have the appearance of a wound in the process of healing, but which never gets there; in fact the "wound" just gets bigger. The similarity is partly due to inflammatory processes which are common to both cancers and healing tissue. Also, it has long been observed that tissues exposed to relentless irritation are prone to cancerous

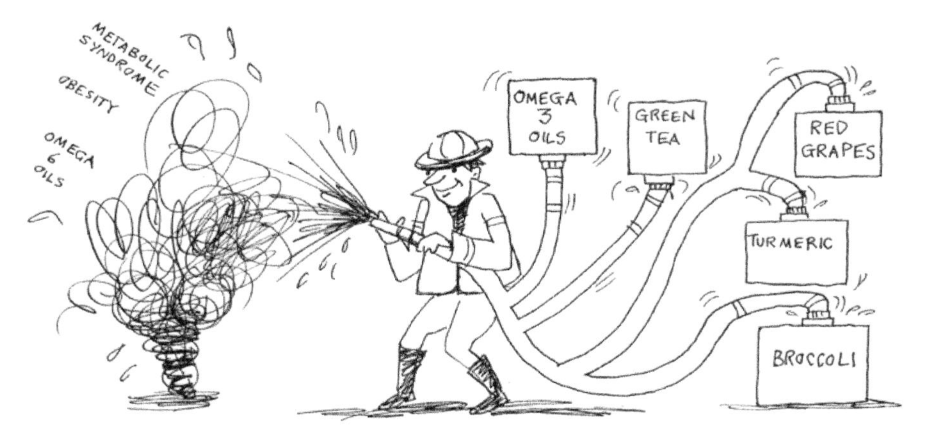

THE FIRE OF INFLAMMATION (FED BY OMEGA 6 OILS, OBESITY AND METABOLIC SYNDROME) CAN BE PUT OUT BY THE WATER OF OMEGA 3 OILS, TURMERIC, GREEN TEA, RED GRAPES AND BROCCOLI.

transformation. For example, this occurs with gastro-oesophageal reflux, inflammatory bowel disease, burn scars, and osteomyelitis.

Non-steroidal anti-inflammatory drugs (NSAIDs) such as aspirin and ibuprofen, are known to protect against some cancers[10].

Inflammation is a normal healthy response to tissue injury. Key elements in healing include cell proliferation (i.e. cell division to replace the lost tissue) and angiogenesis (in-growth of new blood vessels) to provide nutrients to the regenerating tissue. White blood cells and their signalling proteins are part of the process. This is acute (short-term) inflammation and usually results in healing.

However, if the process becomes prolonged, it is termed "chronic" inflammation, and this seems to be where the danger begins. The common elements of both healing and cancer can be seen in the drive for cell division and angiogenesis. In addition, the cells are exposed to the risk of DNA damage (gene mutations) from free radicals which arise in the inflammatory environment, or from toxins or infectious agents that may have been the initial cause of the injury. The opportunity for mutations in DNA is increased because the cells are dividing (replicating their DNA) so frequently. It is easy to see that if these healing cells develop gene mutations, they may permanently retain the drive to proliferate. They find themselves in an environment rich in inflammatory cells and growth factors perfect for supporting them. Furthermore, the factors which enable healthy white blood cells to move through tissue as part of their normal function, may also play a role in tumour migration, invasion and metastases.

There are dozens of plant chemicals which are anti-inflammatory via a host of mechanisms[11]. These include free radical scavenging (prevent antioxidant damage) as well as actions against pro-inflammatory gene expression, enzymes, and inflammatory white blood cells.

For example, curcumin downregulates cyclo-oxygenase (COX-2) which is an inflammatory mediator. Curcumin (turmeric), EGCG (green tea) and resveratrol (red grapes) have been shown to suppress activation of NF-kappa B (a DNA transcription factor involved in inflammation). Sulforaphane blocks the anti-apoptotic effect of certain inflammatory enzymes. Omega 3 fatty acids are anti-inflammatory while Omega 6 are mainly pro-inflammatory. Also, one possible reason that obesity increases cancer risk is the inflammation associated with abdominal adipose tissue in so-called metabolic syndrome, which has been linked to cancer.

Epigenetics

Epigenetics is to do with whether or not a gene is expressed or how it is expressed, and this is determined by factors outside the gene itself. "It's not just in the genes but what we expose them to"[12]. Or stated another way in a Time Magazine article: "Why your DNA isn't your destiny"[13].

I said in the introduction that most cancers are caused by the environment and not genes. Even in patients who have a genetic susceptibility to cancer, food may determine, to some extent, whether or not the cancer gene is expressed in any given individual. For example, in breast cancer, BRCA gene mutations lead to cancer of the breast and

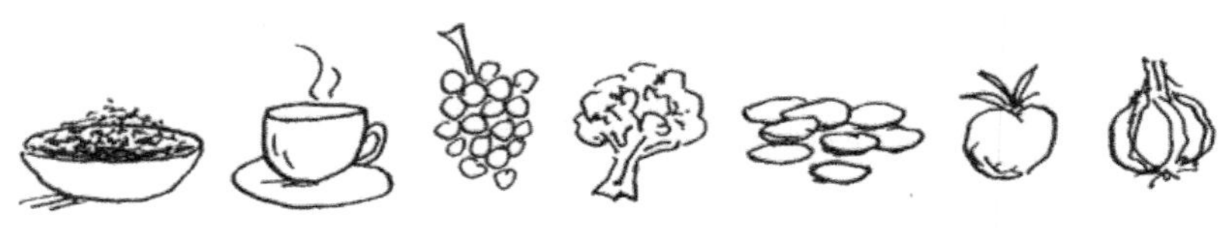

The right food (turmeric, green tea, grapes, broccoli, brazil nuts, tomatoes, garlic) can prevent mutated genes from being expressed.

ovary in many, but not all, of those who carry the mutation. Why? Because there is an interplay between genetics and the environment.

You will have heard of the Human Genome Project in which all the human genes have been mapped out. One of the fascinating findings was that the human genome consists of about 25,000 genes, which is no more than some very simple animals. The much more complicated arrangements of tissues and organs in humans and higher animals is a result of the way in which genes are expressed, rather than just the number of genes present. This has led to the new field of epigenetics.

In the nucleus of the cell, certain stretches of DNA (a gene) are covered by a sleeve of regulating protein that needs to be removed in order for that gene to be read. (By "read" we mean that the gene needs to be exposed in order for the chemical processes to copy the message it contains, and then deliver it for the appropriate effect).

Every cell in the body contains the same DNA, but for a particular cell to develop as a nerve cell or a muscle cell or any other particular cell type, the relevant segment of DNA has to be "read" or "turned on", while the others are not. This is governed by epigenetic factors such as regulatory proteins. These epigenetic regulators are themselves influenced by environmental factors, such as dietary nutrients and chemical exposure.

An example of epigenetics at work is seen in the Agouti mouse, which carries a gene abnormality, causing it to be a yellow colour and very obese. An experiment was done in which some Agouti mouse mothers were given a special diet and others were not. Those with the special diet produced normal lean brown offspring even though they still carried the same abnormal genes as their mothers. The diet had controlled whether the gene was expressed or not[14].

A number of nutrients have been identified as being able to exert such an influence. These include curcumin (turmeric), green tea polyphenols, resveratrol (grapes), sulforaphane (broccoli), selenium, lycopene (tomatoes), genistein (soybeans) and DADS (garlic), among others[15,16].

The point is that there are environmental factors, such as food, which can over-ride underlying genes. Clearly, there is a lot more to learn in this area. In the meantime, if you have a strong family history of cancer or are known to carry a cancer gene, it makes sense to adopt a diet rich in the nutrients that are likely to provide cells with all they need to function optimally, and perhaps prevent the expression of mutated genes.

The Microenvironment

Consider the analogy of the seed and the soil, with the soil being the body's microenvironment and the seed being the cancer. If the soil is not favourable, the seed cannot grow. This is why cancer cells can be present in the body but fail to grow or spread. For example, this is can occur with prostate cancer, papillary cancer of the thyroid, or non-invasive breast cancer. Clearly some cells undergo the first phase of cancer development which is transformation of healthy cells into malignant cells, but then they lack the requirements to grow into a mass or spread to other parts of the body.

The microenvironment (the soil) includes all the cells, blood vessels, cell signalling chemistry, availability of key nutrients, etc. The cancer and the microenvironment each affect the other. Acidity and oxygenation are part of this, and attract much attention in some circles.

It has been observed that in and around a cancer, there tends to be a low level of oxygen and a high level of acid. Some say this is what causes cancer. But is it cause or effect? The opposing view is that the low oxygen and high acid levels are due to the presence of the tumour

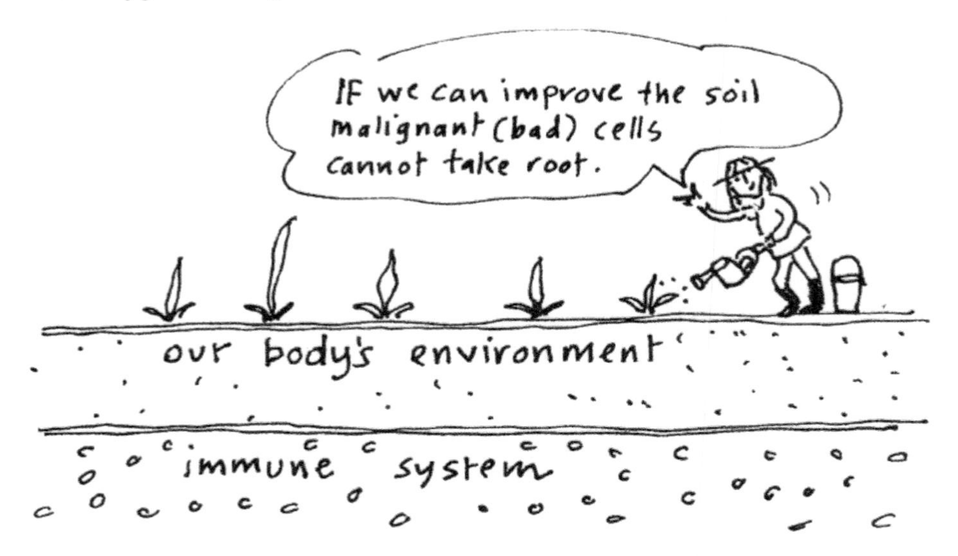

because the cancer cells are using up all the oxygen available, and are now producing acid as a result of the anaerobic metabolism which occurs without oxygen (fermentation instead of glycolysis).

In the first place, a toxic environment favours cancer initiation. Then, as the cancer cells grow into a larger tumour, an increasingly toxic microenvironment develops as a result of the inefficient metabolism and excess waste products. This promotes further gene mutations within the cancer cells. In other words, some of the bad soil is a result of the cancer itself, exacerbating the situation. Whether attempts to change the overall body acidity and oxygenation can be effective, and whether this would then translate into a change in the local tissues around the actual cancer mass, is an area of contention. The blood acidity (pH) operates in a tightly controlled narrow range. You can't easily change blood pH, and nor would you want to. However, some proponents of an alkalinizing diet would say that the acid-buffering system in the background is affected by the acidity of a western diet. They theorize that if this is not addressed, the risk of cancer increases.

In any case, a diet high in vegetables and without excessive meat, dairy and sugar, is on the alkaline side (non-acidic). Such a diet influences cell signalling favourably and provides key nutrients for optimal cell function – i.e. a healthy anticancer microenvironment.

Curcumin: An Example of Phytochemical Effects at Multiple Levels

Curcumin (from turmeric) has been shown to block many phases of cancer progression. This is achieved by either direct molecular interaction, or by blocking the genes which control the production of cancer-favouring chemistry. Curcumin acts to re-assert the normal controls and reverse gene over-expression. Every cell in the body contains every gene, but for any given cell, only some of those genes are supposed to be turned on for the proper function of that cell. Most of the genes are turned off because they are not relevant to that particular cell type, or not needed at that point in time. Cancer cells ignore the rules because they have developed more and more mutations, and are exposed to an increasingly toxic local environment, resulting in the unveiling of vast numbers of inappropriate genes, some of which result in enhanced cancerous properties such as rapid division and invincibility.

This is a list of some of the critical mechanisms that are blocked by curcumin[17-21].

Phase of cancer progression		Mechanism
Cell cycle (process of cell division)	via	cyclins D and E
Cell proliferation (stimulated to grow/divide)	via	EGFR, Her2
Cell survival ("immortal" cancer cell)	via	PBK, AKT pathways
Invasion (of adjacent structures)	via	MMP9, adhesion molecules
Angiogenesis (new feeding blood vessels)	via	VEGF and VEGF receptors, angiopoietin
Metastasis (spread to secondary sites)	via	CXCR-4
Inflammation (chemical messengers promote cancer)	via	NFkB, TNF, IL1/6, COX2, 5LOX

Curcumin also inhibits H pylori bacteria, down-regulates transcription factors and growth factors, inhibits environmental oestrogens, and increases glutathione (an intracellular antioxidant) by inhibiting the enzymes which inhibit it.

19. RESEARCH METHODS AND MAJOR TRIALS

How to Research Food

The abundance of misleading, incomplete or contradictory information is incredible, especially online. Here are some examples.

One writer insists that garlic should not be cooked, but that's not quite true. Another says Brazil nuts are no good if they have already

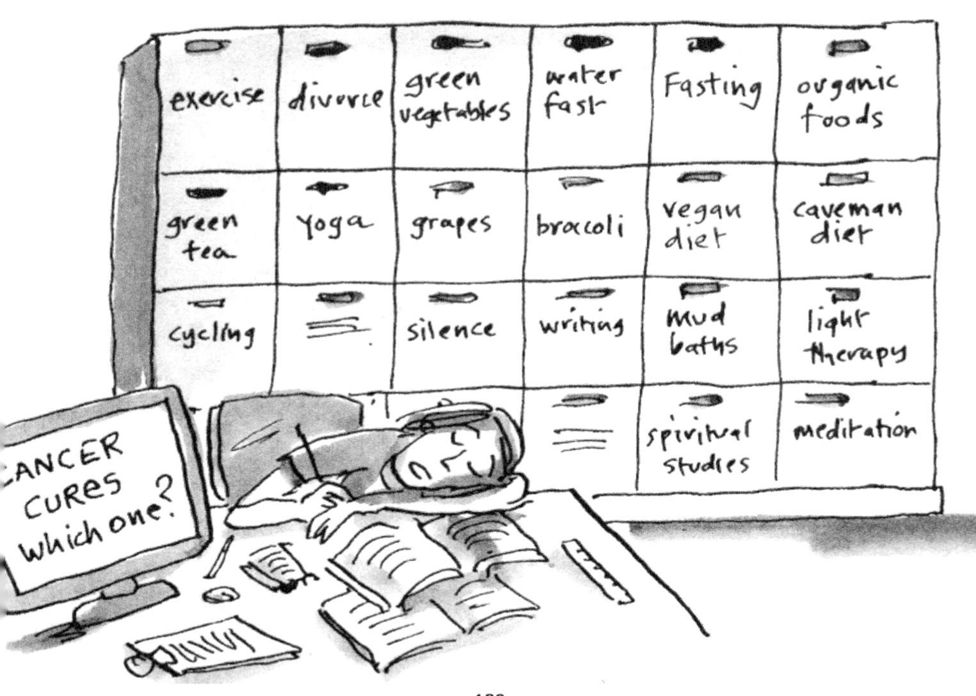

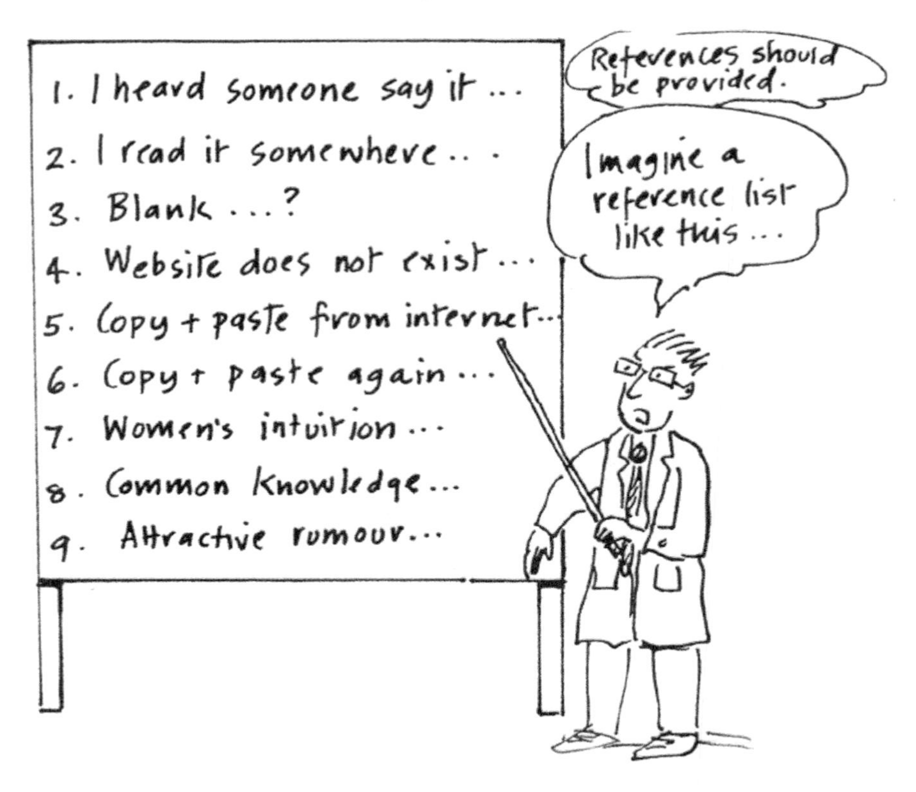

been shelled, but where did that information come from? Mushrooms are advocated against cancer, but few mention that they need to be fresh or stored properly. A commentary concluded that a diet study showed no difference, but it seems to have overlooked key problems. Another says to get your resveratrol from red wine, but do they know that it depends on the grape-growing region?

An online shop was recommended by another online source, saying their selenium product has the best bioavailability, but when I contacted the store, they had no idea what was in their supplement.

All this takes a long time to unravel.

Beware an underlying philosophy that interprets evidence to suit itself. Some writers are convinced that there is an evil "cancer industry" that can't be trusted. They say that a cancer cure is always possible by natural means. This is a nice idea. I wish it were true, but it simply has not been proven. Perhaps some mainstream treatments seem excessive and cause side effects, but often they actually work! The fact is that many patients using unconventional cures deteriorate and die unpleasant deaths. We have to be honest about this. Wishful thinking is not good enough. On the other side of the equation is the sceptic who discounts the value in any lifestyle intervention. He is in danger of throwing the baby out with the bath water. Nutritional information websites from major cancer hospitals tend to be pessimistic with regard to the anticancer effects of food. We need to see beyond any bias, including our own.

If there are no sources quoted in an article or book, be cautious. Further searching may locate the original source. When this is read, it may be obvious that the claim has been overstated. For example, a recent webpage headline shouted that a certain plant extract cured breast cancer. When I traced the publication, it was just a small rodent study. The fact that this was not a human study had been omitted. Although news articles or press releases relating to research may overstate a point, they will often direct you to a useful source. On the other hand, health and wellness sites will frequently make a lot of statements with no references. They may have just copied the information from another site or a popular book. Even if it is well written, be slow to believe until you see confirmation elsewhere (and not just another requote of the same unsourced material!). Some writers betray their lack of scientific education by making statements that they clearly don't understand. A reader with a science education can often tell immediately if a site is not to be trusted.

If you have found a claim, such as a plant food which has anticancer potential, you can search for it on PubMed which is online. This will show a list of published journal articles on the subject, and the abstract (summary) is nearly always available. These articles are written by scientists and are usually peer-reviewed. This means that the work was checked by reputable people in the same field to verify that the standard of research and writing is acceptable. The full article may be free online, but some articles can be difficult to obtain. At least you will learn something from the abstract. Often there are review articles which summarize the best research and provide references to scores of relevant articles.

This is the kind of process I have applied over a number of years, leading me to hundreds of scientific articles. I have read widely to give a fair hearing to alternative ideas, and to look for new information. I ask if there is enough evidence to make us change what we do. What are the facts?

Types of Studies and Trials

Anecdotes and case studies

Often, a potential treatment will start as an observation that a single person had some benefit from an intervention. This is termed a case report. (If it is poorly documented or unverified, it may be termed "anecdotal"- i.e. simply an account of an incident.) A group of similar cases is called a series. A particular observation may be made on a larger number of people perhaps in a geographic area. This may lead to formal population studies to see if an association can be made that is strong enough to propose cause and effect.

Animal models and cancer cell cultures

Animal studies can be done to explore a hypothesis, or to see if an observed effect is reproducible. Human cancer cells can be transferred to rodents, after which cancer growth and spread are measured. However, animals do have slightly different systems to humans. Cancer cures in animals will not necessarily result in a cure for humans, but the physiology and biochemistry can be analysed to see why it works. Promising results indicate that the treatment should be investigated further.

Cells can be taken from human cancers and grown in the laboratory. These cancer cell cultures can then be subjected to treatments and once again the microscopic and biochemical effects recorded.

(Frequently at this point, if a natural substance has been the subject of investigation, it will be modified to see if it can be made more powerful. This also means that, unlike the naturally occurring substance, it can be patented and marketed by a drug company. This causes a number of potential problems. Firstly, the modification may also cause side effects not seen with the unaltered substance. Secondly, attempts to isolate the active ingredient means that other effective components of the whole food, for example, will be lost, along with any synergy between the elements.)

Case control studies

A case control study is one in which a group of people with a disease are compared to a group who don't have it. The factor under study is something thought to influence the risk of having the disease. For example, we can examine cancer patients (the "cases") and show that they have lower levels of a certain phytochemical in their body compared to a group of people who don't have cancer (the "controls"). This would suggest (but does not prove) that the particular phytochemical reduces the risk of cancer.

Cohort studies

A cohort study differs because no-one in the study has the disease yet. However, some of the participants are known to be exposed to the factor under study, while the others are not. Over time, when the disease appears, we can see if it is more or less likely to happen to the ones exposed to the factor under trial. For example, we can take a large group and record who in the group eats the most garlic. Over time, if the garlic eaters get less cancer than the non-eaters, a causal link may be postulated. The cohort may be one large group with similar background characteristics, and after a time, subgroups within the cohort are compared for various risk factors. Or there may be two cohorts from the start, one with the risk factor (or protective factor) and one without it. At the end of the time period the incidence of cancer is compared. Cohort studies collect data before the disease develops (prospective) which is more reliable than case control studies which look back (retrospective) to identify correlation.

Findings from case control and cohort studies are not considered to be as convincing as randomized control trials, because there is more potential for unrecognized biases. For this reason, such studies are able to identify an association between diet and cancer but cannot absolutely prove a causal relationship. Case control and cohort studies are the methods commonly used to assess nutrition because the nature of diet does not lend itself to clinical trials. Diet cannot be "controlled".

Clinical trials

The clinical trial applies the principles of a scientific experiment in which subjects are randomized to one intervention (treatment) or another, or to be in a control group. This is the best way to demonstrate cause and effect, but is only valid if the intervention can be reliably and accurately applied. In food terms, this would entail a strict diet with no deviation whatsoever, keeping food sources, quantity, preparation, combinations, etc all absolutely uniform. This is impossible in practice. On the other hand, typical medical treatments, such as a tablet or a surgical procedure, can be more distinctly applied and monitored, although many problems can still arise to spoil the results.

The RCT (Randomized controlled trial)

A randomized controlled trial takes two or more groups and randomly assigns a treatment with each group receiving a different treatment (or one group may receive a placebo). Results are compared after an interval. This is considered the most accurate type of trial. It is even more convincing if a number of RCTs look at the same question and arrive at the same conclusion (a meta-analysis).

However, even RCTs can be wrong. Although this type of trial is usually considered to be very reliable, there are many potential flaws. Also, it can be difficult to eliminate conflicts of interest (or "vested interests") if trial funding comes from the drug company that is manufacturing the product, or if the researchers are desperate for good results. Statistical analysis may be done in a way that suits the desired outcome. A negative result is as important as a positive one, but unfavourable results are frequently not published[1]. RCTs are not perfect and if the results are not able to be reproduced, they remain under question.

Do We Need To Wait for an RCT?

In the green tea section, I selected some studies showing a favourable effect. Even so, it must be acknowledged that many reviewers conclude that there is not enough evidence. The Cochrane Review of 51 studies on green tea, reported conflicting results due to confounding variables[2].

However, when animal studies, cell culture studies, epidemiology, and many clinical trials show a benefit, how can they be ignored? It is very difficult, if not impossible to absolutely eliminate any confounding variables when dealing with nutrition. So of course there are going to be some conflicting results. Food is complex - sources,

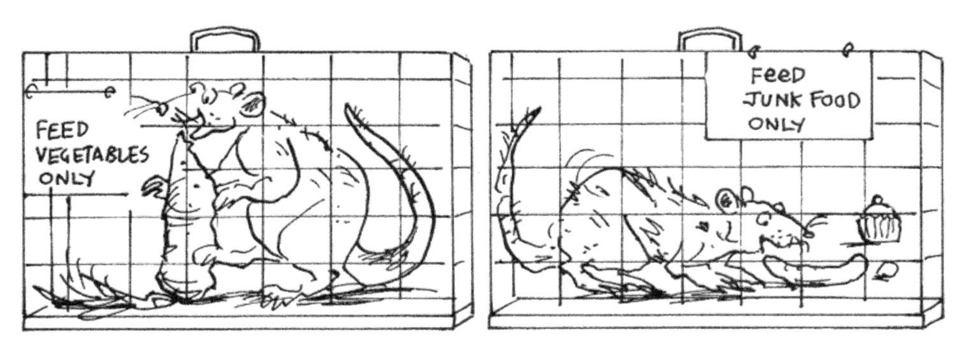

THIS EXPERIMENT MIGHT BE TRIED ON RATS, BUT YOU CAN'T DO IT WITH HUMANS.

preparation, doses, synergy with other foods, etc will vary, as will other lifestyle factors. People are inconsistent in what they eat (or drink) and unreliable in what they report. The trials will never be good enough, and the reviewers may never be satisfied.

It follows that large cancer organizations and journal editors will nearly always say that the evidence is uncertain and more trials are needed, partly because they don't want to be held accountable for any statements seen as too optimistic.

Why not recommend good food? What is there to lose? There are no side effects! Nutrition is safe and cheap. And healthy!

Some people seem to be bound by the insistence on randomized controlled trials, always concluding that they are waiting for one. Well they may be waiting forever. Besides, RCTs are not perfect either. The books "It's Great! Oops, No It Isn't" by Ronald Gauch[3] and "Bad Pharma" by Ben Goldacre[1] explain why clinical research can't guarantee the right medical answers. People seem to have forgotten that accurate observation, even of a single case, is still useful information. How many times would you watch a child being hit by a car before you concluded that safe crossings are needed? Did they do a randomized trial? I know that trials of that sort are unethical, but do you see the point?

Observational studies do carry weight, and logical deductions play an important role. This is particularly so in the study of diet and cancer because the field is so complicated. Many variables are at play and simply cannot be controlled. Therefore, we do need to consider the relevance of trends, and look at the mounting weight of evidence coming from many angles.

Consider the animal studies providing "proof of principle", and the multitude of anticancer mechanisms of action at cellular and molecular levels identified in the laboratory. Unfortunately this information hasn't made it into the text books, and we have been told to keep waiting for that RCT.

Some of the green tea studies I have described were rejected as not good enough by the Cochrane Review, but if the findings are by chance, why don't we see an equal number showing that green tea increases cancer risk? Instead, a positive effect is seen over and over again. As with other dietary cancer preventers, the volume of evidence from so many sources becomes compelling.

Did you know that smoking as a cause of lung cancer has never been tested in a RCT? This is because you can't randomize subjects to smoke cigarettes or not (and you can't make people conform to a certain diet, either). The evidence for a link between smoking and cancer came from cohort and case control studies, but for years it was not believed! Are we going to make the same mistake with diet and cancer?

Serum Rhubarb

In medical practice, we jokingly use the term "serum rhubarb" (which doesn't exist) to refer to obscure tests ordered by only the most detailed and fussy physician. Now, it seems, we can actually do a blood test for vegetable levels.

When looking for a reduction in cancer from vegetables, not all studies have produced convincing results. This is at least in part because they rely on questionnaires. How reliable can it be? Do you remember exactly what you have eaten for the last five years? To address this, some have looked at the carotene levels in blood samples to give a more accurate measure of the quantity of vegetables consumed.

In a cohort of women from New York, no difference in breast cancer rates was seen when the answers to a dietary questionnaire were used[4]. However, when actual blood levels of carotenoids were tested, a difference became apparent[5]. This strongly suggests that participants had not accurately remembered or reported what they had eaten. A systematic review concurs with this conclusion[6].

A study of women who had already had a breast cancer, also measured total carotenoids in blood samples[7]. Those with the highest levels (top quarter) had a reduced risk (43% less) for developing a new or recurrent breast cancer, compared to those with the lowest levels.

In another one, alpha-carotene in the blood was measured. Those with the highest levels were much less likely to die from cancer, especially from aerodigestive cancers, than those with the lowest levels[8].

Swiss researchers observed that not only did low blood levels of beta-carotene and vitamin A increase the risk of having lung or gastric cancer, but also increased the risk of death from any form of cancer[9]. Likewise, a Chinese study showed that higher blood carotenes were associated with a reduction in gastric cancers[10].

Blood levels of carotenoids are considered to be a "marker" of intake of fruit and vegetables in general. People who have a lot of carotene in their blood have usually been eating lots of other vegetables as well. In other words, a reduction in cancer is probably not just due to the carotenes, but also from the other phytochemicals. For example, cruciferous vegetables like broccoli not only contain carotenes, but also the anticancer sulforaphane and indole-3-carbinol.

Major Population Trials and Studies

There have been many attempts to answer the question of whether diet influences cancer. Listed below are the key ones, with a quote from the reported conclusions. Some have negative findings and there are possible reasons for this, as discussed afterwards. It could be said that in light of the difficulties with these kinds of studies, the fact that any positive differences are found at all strengthens the case for diet against cancer.

In (mainly) chronological order:

1. Iowa Women's Health Study: Vegetables, fruit and colon cancer Am J Epidemiol 1994[11]

   Consumption of garlic, all vegetables and fibre were each inversely associated with risk, when uppermost and lowermost quartiles were compared.

2. WINS (Women's Intervention Nutrition Study): Dietary fat and breast cancer. J NCI 2006[12]

   Conclusion: A lifestyle intervention reducing dietary fat intake, with modest influence on body weight, may improve relapse-free survival of breast cancer patients receiving conventional cancer management.

   Also note that a report on this trial was given at the 2005 meeting of ASCO (American Society of Clinical Oncology) stating that the diet resulted in significant reduction of breast cancer recurrence, especially for oestrogen negative cancers.

3. WHI (Women's Health Initiative): Low fat diet and breast cancer. JAMA 2006[13]

   Among post-menopausal women, a low-fat dietary pattern did not result in a statistically significant reduction in invasive breast cancer risk over an 8.1 year average follow-up period (although a favourable trend was observed).

4. WHEL (Women's Healthy Eating and Living randomized trial) JAMA 2007[14]

   Among survivors of early stage breast cancer, adoption of a diet that was very high in vegetables, fruit, and fiber and low in fat did not reduce additional breast cancer events or mortality during a 7.3 year follow-up period.

5. Plasma carotenoids and recurrence-free survival in breast cancer (WHEL subset). J Clin Oncol 2005[7]

   This study supports findings that have linked increased vegetable and fruit intake with greater likelihood of recurrence-free survival in early-stage breast cancer.

6. Serum alpha-carotene and risk of death among US adults. Arch Int Med 2011[8]

   Serum alpha-carotene concentrations were inversely associated with risk of death from all causes, including cancer. These findings support increasing fruit and vegetable consumption as a means of preventing premature death.

7. EPIC (European Prospective Investigation into Cancer and Nutrition Study). Various publications 2002-2005, ongoing[15-17]

The combination of four dietary factors (i.e. fibre, fish, red meat and processed meats) plays a major role in colorectal cancer aetiology in addition to alcohol intake, obesity and low physical activity. Consumption of fruit and vegetables was not associated with risk of cancer of the breast, ovary or prostate (although garlic and onions may exert a beneficial effect).

8. Greek EPIC cohort: Mediterranean diet and cancer. BJ Cancer 2008[18]

Just two (of nine) elements of the Mediterranean diet reduced cancer incidence by 12%. When increased to six items per day, cancer risk falls by 22%.

9. Asian American Women: Dietary patterns and breast cancer risk. Am J Clin Nutr 2009[19]

Results suggest that a diet characterized by a low intake of meat/starches and a high intake of legumes is associated with a reduced risk of breast cancer in Asian Americans.

10. Black Women's Health Study: Fruit and vegetable intake in relation to risk of breast cancer. Am J Epid 2010[20]

Fruit and vegetable intakes were not significantly associated with overall risk of breast cancer. However, total vegetable consumption was associated with a decreased risk of oestrogen receptor-negative breast cancer. In addition, there was some evidence of inverse associations (i.e. trend) with breast cancer risk overall for cruciferous vegetable intake and for carrot intake.

11. Danish cohort study on lifestyle and colorectal cancer. BMJ 2010[21]

Adherence to the recommendations for physical activity, waist circumference, smoking, alcohol intake, and diet may reduce colorectal cancer risk considerably, and in this population, 23% of the cases might be attributable to lack of adherence to the five lifestyle recommendations.

12. Nurses' Health Study: Dietary fat and fiber in relation to risk of breast cancer. JAMA 2011[22]

These data provide evidence against both an adverse influence of fat intake and a protective effect of fibre consumption by middle-aged women on breast cancer incidence over eight years.

Why don't the major trials always show a benefit of food against cancer?

- Self-reporting of food consumed is unreliable, as evidenced by serum carotenoid tests, and by failure to lose weight despite supposedly lower caloric intake.
- The group which is supposed to modify their diet becomes slack, and the group which is not supposed to make changes tends to do so anyway because they become conscious of their food once they are in the trial. Thus the diets of the two groups actually become very similar over time, which means that a benefit from diet won't be demonstrable.
- Not all vegetables are the same. Vegetable types, sources, method of preparation, etc are usually not taken into account.
- Not all fats are the same. Animal fat, polyunsaturated fat, Omega 3 or 6 dominance, and trans-fats all have different implications with regard to cancer, but this distinction is not made in the trials.
- Fat is not really the issue. A low fat diet will not necessarily contain any more cancer-fighting phytochemicals than a diet with more fat. Fat consumption will be a problem if it causes obesity which carries a cancer risk. Low fat eaters may substitute with carbohydrates which may carry a greater cancer risk either directly or via obesity.
- Even those with the "best" dietary habits will often have a relatively poor diet. For example, in one study, the top group was anyone who ate over 309g of vegetables per day. That really isn't very much. A capsicum weighs 100g. A good serving of broccoli and two large carrots comes to 400g. How can they expect to see any difference when they are comparing poor diets to diets that are only marginally better?
- Cancer usually takes years to develop, and specific foods differ in their roles in cancer initiation, growth or metastases. The change in diet may be too late for older participants who still reap the consequences of all the preceding years. Follow-up of even 7 or 8 years may not be enough to see the full effects of a better diet.

Look at the statements below that strongly favour the role of food against cancer. There is a disparity between them and the lukewarm conclusions of the major dietary studies listed on the preceding page. The statements below are quite clear that diet is a factor that can prevent cancer, but some of the big studies above say that diet makes little or no difference. The weight of evidence would suggest that it is the negative studies which are likely to be flawed.

Reports addressing lifestyle and cancer risk: Future burden and cancer prevention

1. Estimating the burden of cancer in Australia. MJA 2012[23]
   "Our projections suggest that there will be about 170,000 Australians diagnosed with cancer in 2025. Almost 43,000 of these cancers could be prevented through improvements to diet and physical activity levels, including through their impact on obesity."

2. Cancer prevention and early detection facts and figures (American Cancer Society)[24].
   "Approximately one-third of the 571,950 deaths expected to occur in 2011 (in the USA) are attributed to poor nutrition, physical inactivity, overweight, and obesity."

3. The fraction of cancer attributable to lifestyle and environmental factors in the UK in 2010. B J Cancer 2011[25]

"Looking at all the evidence, it's clear that around 40 percent of all cancers are caused by things we mostly have the power to change."[26]

Research Notes: Biology, Chemistry and Studies

For each topic that follows, technical or scientific detail is provided to complement the earlier chapters.

As I stated in the introduction, I am happy to acknowledge that while we do see some negative or neutral studies, I have focused on those which demonstrate the positive results of nutrients against cancer. This approach is based on what I would consider to be adequate proof of mechanism, proof of concept and convincing statistical associations, as seen in laboratory work and epidemiological observations.

20. BROCCOLI AND THE CRUCIFERS RESEARCH NOTES

Cruciferous Chemistry

Broccoli contains at least 17 nutrients called glucosides. The main ones we're interested in are glucoraphain (GRP) and glucobrassicin. These can act independently, but all 17 also work synergistically, meaning an even greater benefit than the added effects of each one on its own.

Sulforaphane Production: the Importance of Myrosinase

The GRP is located in the main substance (cytoplasm) of the cell and has no special beneficial effects as it is. However, when exposed to an enzyme called myrosinase, the GRP is converted to **sulforaphane (SF)**, an isothiocyanate (ITC). The myrosinase is contained within the cell wall. When the plant is chewed, the cell wall is broken, allowing the myrosinase to escape and come into contact with the GRP, leading to the production of SF. This has important implications.

A purified GRP supplement from broccoli would do you no good because myrosinase is required to generate SF[4]. Also, myrosinase is destroyed by overcooking[8]. If broccoli is overcooked, a small amount of GRP will still be converted to SF because the bacteria in the lower bowel possess some myrosinase-like activity[18]. Eating raw broccoli (must be chewed well) results in ten times as much SF as when it is excessively cooked[19]. However, myrosinase is not significantly reduced by lightly steaming the vegetable. If broccoli is more thoroughly cooked, some myrosinase can be provided by simultaneous consumption of other plants from the crucifer family[4]. This is an opportunity to spice up your meal with mustard, horseradish or wasabi[20].

Broccoli Sprouts

Phytochemicals in nature protect the plant from potential environmental toxins and from free radicals released during photosynthesis. Perhaps the plant is most vulnerable when it is small, which may explain why the concentration of these protective chemicals is greater in sprouts compared to the mature plant. Broccoli seeds contain the highest amount of GRP but should not be eaten because they also contain erucic acid which may cause heart damage if consumed in very large amounts (unproven). However, the erucic acid disappears when the seeds sprout[21,22]. Broccoli sprouts retain exceptionally high levels of GRP[6]. You would need to eat 20 to 50 times more mature broccoli to obtain as much GRP as in sprouts. Sprouts have been used to achieve high levels of SF in a number of studies. However, it should be noted that 90% of the glucosides in sprouts are in the form of GRP (which becomes SF). Sprouts contain very little of the glucoside needed to produce indoles, which are also important.

Indoles

The main indole is **indole-3-carbinol (I3C)** which comes from glucobrassicin (as opposed to GRP). Once again, the I3C is not particularly active unless two of these molecules join together to form diindolylmethane (DIM), which results in most of the anticancer actions of the indole chemicals. DIM is not formed readily in a neutral environment, but does so in an acidic environment, such as the stomach[23]. Hence, the quantities of I3C required for a useful effect may be less after oral ingestion (which exposes it to stomach acid) compared to what is needed in laboratory experiments.

As mentioned, you won't get much I3C from sprouts, so for the benefits of the indoles, mature broccoli should be eaten. In particular, this applies to the anti-oestrogen effects important in preventing breast cancer.

Mechanism of Action

SF and I3C work differently (although there is some overlap).

Sulforaphane (SF)

1. Induction of enzymes via gene expression[24]

What you eat can actually affect which genes are expressed. This to do with "epigenetics" which is the study of how and when a gene is expressed. We now know that the cellular environment (including phytochemicals) affects genes.

SF induces expression of Phase 2 genes.

A word of explanation about genes and enzymes: Genes carry the code or instructions for making proteins. Enzymes are a kind of protein. Enzymes speed up chemical reactions, or in effect cause chemical reactions that would otherwise have happened too slowly to be of any use.

Phase 1 and Phase 2 enzymes are for detoxification - i.e. removing harmful chemicals. Phase 1 converts foreign substances into a form which the Phase 2 enzymes can work on. Phase 2 converts the Phase 1 products into less reactive

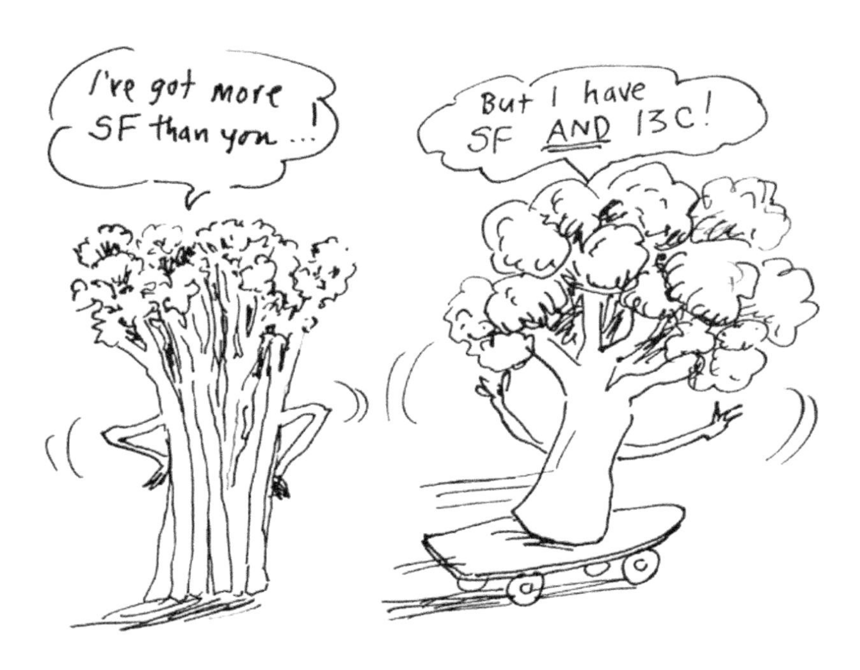

chemicals which can then be easily excreted from the cell and then out of the body. These Phase 1 and 2 reactions are a way of removing carcinogens (substances that cause cancer). These phases are part of the antioxidant system. You will be familiar with the idea that food containing antioxidants is good for you, and helps prevent cancer. SF particularly induces Phase 2 genes (e.g. for glutathione-s-transferase) but also has a positive effect on Phase 1 genes (e.g. cytochrome p450).

Specifically, SF is taken into the cell where it activates a transcription factor called Nrf2. This moves into the cell nucleus where it lines up with a particular section of the gene which makes Phase 2 enzymes. The section it lines up with is called the "antioxidant response element", which is in the promoter region of the gene, and so the gene is turned on.

Here we have a plant nutrient (SF) which doesn't just work directly as an antioxidant, but actually causes expression of genes which turn on a whole production of enzyme proteins - i.e. a huge multiplier effect equivalent to thousands of individual antioxidant molecules. Without this happening, the cell we are talking about would not be able to protect itself from damage. Damage leads to changes which can turn the cell into a cancerous one.

Wow! If your cells are exposed to any toxic rubbish that could lead to cancer, those protective mechanisms clear it out before the trouble begins. And if you have some SF in your system, it is put into high gear. Even though the SF itself may only be at high levels in your blood for a few hours, the ongoing antioxidant effect lasts for three days.

2. Cell cycle arrest

When SF is applied to cancer cells in the lab, the dividing cell is seen to be stuck halfway through the cell cycle[25]. It has stopped dividing! This is how some chemotherapy drugs work.

3. Apoptosis

Apoptosis is also called programmed cell death. SF promotes appropriate apoptosis. Broccoli is synergistic with turmeric in causing apoptosis in prostate cancer cells[26], while leaving normal cells unaffected[27].

4. Angiogenesis

SF reduces the formation of new capillaries in lab experiments. It does this in a number of ways, one of which is by interfering with vascular endothelial growth factor (VEGF)[25].

5. Invasion and metastasis[25]

Cancer becomes life-threatening when it progresses beyond a self-contained lump and invades into surrounding tissue, or breaks into blood vessels or lymph channels and moves through them to another part of the body (metastasis).

Cancer cell movement through the wall of a blood vessel or other structure is called migration. In the laboratory, SF has been shown to inhibit cell migration. Broccoli and watercress extracts suppress enzymes which are involved in invasiveness of breast cancer cells. In mice, melanoma cells injected into the blood stream usually settle in the lungs and form cancerous lumps but when SF was given at a low dose, the lung nodule formation was inhibited. This effect was not from the SF directly killing the cancer cells, but by blocking the enzymes which are required for invasion.

Indoles - Mechanism of Action of I3C

1. Induces Phase 1 and 2 enzymes to remove carcinogenic substances including those in tobacco smoke and in cooked food[27].
2. Blocks androgen (male hormone) receptors in prostate cancer cells[28].
3. Effects on oestrogen (mainly applies to oestrogen-sensitive tissue such as breast and uterus).

Oestrogen metabolism

Normally oestrogen (oestradiol, E2) is metabolized (changed) to other forms including 2-hydroxyoestrone (2OH-E1) and 16alpha-hydroxyoestrone (16aOH-E1). The "16alpha" (bad) has greater oestrogenic activity and therefore increases breast cancer risk or growth. I3C in crucifer vegetables shifts metabolism to favour production of 2OH-E1 (good), which has the opposite (protective) effect[29,30].

Oestrogen receptor blockade

Oestrogen is essentially a growth-promoting hormone and regulates many genes that are involved in cell proliferation. I3C blocks oestrogen from activating the oestrogen receptor and hence blocks the tendency for that cell to become cancerous (or to grow and divide if it is already a cancer cell). This effect also occurs via the BRCA1 protein. I3C and BRCA1 inhibit the receptor function synergistically. Furthermore, I3C upregulates (magnifies) BRCA1[31].

Note: You have probably heard of BRCA (stands for BReast CAncer) as a genetic cause of breast cancer. Also see Epigenetics p.124. The normal BRCA gene is a tumour suppressor (good), so when the gene is mutated, the suppressor effect is lost. It is a mutation of the normal BRCA which leads to cancer. When patients are referred to as "having the BRCA gene", we really should say "a mutated BRCA gene".

I3C is synergistic with the drug tamoxifen in inhibiting growth of breast cancer cells.

4. Other effects of I3C[31]:

Detoxifies carcinogens.

Induces apoptosis.

Is an antioxidant.

Induces p21 expression which inhibits proliferation, and produces G1/S stasis (cytostatic)[9].

Synergizes with the drug Paclitaxel to induce apoptosis in Her 2 positive breast cancer cells[32].

Other crucifers may have additional specific mechanisms of action.

For example, watercress contains phenyethyl isothiocyanate (PE-ITC) which prevents angiogenesis by blocking HIF (hypoxia induction factor) produced by the tumour[33]. PE-ITC also restores p53 which allows apoptosis to occur[34].

Research Papers

There are scores of papers with favourable results in animal studies and cell cultures which I have not listed. Below are summaries of some studies involving humans. There are many others.

1. Indole-3-Carbinol (I3C) and colon cancer, in Annals of Oncology, 2007[35]

   Volunteers were given I3C as an oral dose of 400mg per day for three months. When their blood was sampled and the serum applied to cancer cells in a lab dish, there was a significant decrease in proliferation of the cancer cells.

2. Bladder cancer recurrence (and death), USA, in Cancer Epid Biomarkers Prev, 2010[36]

   239 patients with bladder cancer were followed up for an average of eight years. 101 of them died from the cancer during this period. Analysis was made of the amount of raw broccoli which was eaten.

   184 who ate <1 serve/mth – 85/184 died = 46%
   55 who ate > 1 serve/mth – 16/55 died = 29%

   When the results were adjusted to take into account other risk factors, statistically, the risk of dying if you ate more broccoli compared to less broccoli was 0.43 i.e. the relative risk of dying from cancer was more than halved! In terms of absolute risk, the benefit of eating raw broccoli would be greater than 20% (many orthodox cancer treatments struggle to reach these figures).

   The average amount eaten in the favourable group was about four servings per month.

3. Crucifer intake and cancer risk, Europe, in Annals of Oncology, 2012[17]

   12,449 patients with cancer of many different types, compared to 11,429 controls (other hospital patients without cancer).

Diet was analysed for the preceding 2 years for both groups. Those with cancer were less likely to have eaten crucifer vegetables. For those who ate one or more portions of crucifers/wk, the odds ratio for a breast or colon cancer diagnosis was 0.83 i.e. 17% less likely to be diagnosed with that cancer.

Risk was also reduced for cancers of the oral cavity, pharynx, oesophagus and kidney.

4. Crucifers and breast cancer #1, in Cancer Research, 2003[9]

Shanghai Breast Cancer Survivors (sub-study)

337 breast cancer cases were compared to 337 controls (without breast cancer but matched to the cancer patients in every other way).

Urine SF was measured in both groups, and the groups divided into quartiles (highest urine levels down to lowest). Dietary intake of crucifers assessed by questionnaire.

Those without breast cancer were found to have more SF in their urine. More SF in the urine means more in the blood which means more in the diet (on average, i.e. allowing for variations in individual metabolism). In fact, the participants in the highest quartile (of urinary SF) were 50% less likely to be diagnosed with breast cancer compared to the lowest quartile.

The statistical risk reduction indicated by "odds ratios" (OR) in these studies can be a little difficult to conceptualize, but clearly a plot of the data shows an even distribution in the unaffected people compared to an obvious skew to low SF levels in the cancer patients.

5. Crucifers and breast cancer #2 at the American Association for Cancer Research Annual Meeting, 2012[15]

Shanghai Breast Cancer Survivors (sub-study), presented in 2012 but not yet published.

4866 breast cancer patients. Crucifer intake was measured and the patients followed for the first three years.

Patients with the highest quartile of crucifer intake had a cancer death rate 62% less than those in the lowest quartile. This a relative risk reduction. I could not access the raw data, but it would equate to an absolute survival benefit of about 5%, which is actually very good over such a short period. (Chemotherapy may be given even for a 1 or 2% survival benefit over 10 years.)

6. Crucifers and breast cancer #3, in JAMA, 2001[16]

Swedish study comparing 2832 breast cancer patients to 2650 controls.

Relative risk of developing breast cancer was reduced by 42% for the top decile (median 1.5 serves/day) or by 24% for the top quartile (median 1.1 serves per day), compared to those who ate the least (virtually none).

Note: The results from #5 and #6 above were in contrast to neutral findings from "pooled results" which did not show a statistical benefit.

7. Broccoli and skin cancer, in Proceeds of National Academy of Science, 2007[37]

SF was extracted from broccoli sprouts and applied to human skin. The skin was then exposed to UV light. Erythema (redness) was then measured as a sign of skin damage. Erythema was decreased by 37% in those who had the SF applied.

(In similar studies done with rats, skin cancers were reduced by half when SF was applied.)

21. BERRIES RESEARCH NOTES

Anticancer effects of black raspberries in the rat oesophagus.

As detailed in: Stoner GD. Foodstuffs for Preventing Cancer: The Preclinical and Clinical Development of Berries. Cancer Prev Res (Phila). 2009 Mar;2(3):187-194

Four Key Anticancer Mechanisms

		Inhibits, blocks or reduces
1.	Inhibits cell proliferation	PCNA, Ki-67, AP-1, ERK1/2
2.	Suppresses inflammation	COX-2, PGE-2, iNOS, NF-kB, CD45
3.	Blocks angiogenesis	VEGF-1, HIF-1a, microvessel density
		Increases, promotes or enhances
4.	Promotes apoptosis	TUNEL, Bax, Caspase-3

PCNA	proliferating cell nuclear antigen
Ki-67	protein marker of active cell proliferation
AP-1	activator protein-1, a transcription factor regulating gene expression

ERK	extracellular-signal-regulated kinases (regulate cell division)
COX-2	cyclo-oxygenase-2
PGE-2	prostaglandin E2
iNOS	inducible nitric oxide synthase
NF-kB	nuclear factor kappa B
CD45	leukocyte common antigen
VEGF-1	vascular endothelial growth factor-1
HIF-1a	hypoxia-inducible factor-1alpha
TUNEL	terminal deoxynucleotidyl transferase dUTP nick end labelling
Bax	a pro-apoptotic protein
Caspase-3	interacts with other caspase enzymes in apoptosis pathway

22. TURMERIC RESEARCH NOTES

Mechanism of Action *(see p.127)*

Effect on Chemotherapy

In most cases, curcumin may well increase the effectiveness of chemotherapy, and may even work against cancers which have become resistant to chemotherapy. Chemo-resistance is when chemo initially works well, but if the cancer reappears or starts growing again, this time the chemo does nothing against it. Chemo-resistance may be due to NFkB[9], which is turned on by most chemo drugs. Curcumin blocks NFkB making the cancer cells susceptible to apoptosis again (NFkB stands for nuclear factor kappa-light chain-enhancer of activated B cells. It is a protein complex that is part of many cell signalling pathways, controlling DNA transcription and leading to a variety of cell responses). They regain their "forgotten" apoptosis. The cancer cells develop a multidrug-resistant pathway that is blocked by curcumin, thus restoring chemosensitivity. This may be in part due to curcumin's interference with the "P-gp" cell membrane pump, often over-expressed in cancer cells, which expels chemo agents from the cell[10].

Curcumin sensitizes ovarian cancer to cisplatin[11], and has been claimed to be synergistic with taxol[12].

However, laboratory work suggests that curcumin may reduce the effectiveness of certain types of chemotherapy. These include cyclophosphamide[13] and possibly doxorubicin (conflicting opinions). It would seem best to avoid curcumin while on these drugs.

Bioavailability[14]

Poor bioavailability is the main problem with curcumin. However, there are ways to deal with it.

Low blood levels of curcumin after eating it are due to poor absorption in the bowel, rapid metabolism (conversion to less active forms by conjugation with glucose or sulfur), and rapid elimination (removal from the body by the liver).

Experimental approaches that involve liposomes, nanoparticles and structural analogues are being explored, but in the meantime, bioavailability can be improved by the simple use of pepper and oil.

Black pepper contains piperine. This is a common addition to meals that already have turmeric as an ingredient, especially curry. Participants in one study were given 2g of curcumin and 20mg of piperine, and the bioavailability of curcumin increased 2000% (i.e. 20 times)[15]. Piperine blocks the glucuronidation of curcumin (conversion to a less active form). Not only that, but piperine independently reduces cancer in animal studies[16]. Furthermore, either alone or with curcumin, piperine inhibits breast cancer stem cell renewal (a cause of cancer recurrence)[17].

Another way to improve blood levels is to combine curcumin with oil[14]. Curcumin dissolves very poorly in water, but is more soluble in fat. Adding oil to turmeric powder is said to increase absorption by eight times. Also, mixing it with oil means that once it passes through the intestinal wall, it enters the lymph channels rather than the bloodstream. Lymph does not travel to the liver but goes into the main blood circulation via lymph channels, and so avoids liver breakdown, at least initially. Of course, all the blood volume eventually enters the liver but at least the curcumin is avoiding "first pass metabolism".

Curcumin is not destroyed by cooking. On the contrary, bioavailability of curcumin is improved by heating (e.g. in the oil and pepper mixture).

Dose

In one colon cancer trial, the dose of curcumin was 3600mg per day, while in another it was 480mg (with quercetin). However, bowel wall tissue levels of curcumin will be much higher than in any other tissues because direct contact occurs (i.e. does not depend on good blood levels being achieved).

Makers of supplements suggest 250-400mg twice a day.

In the first study to show the benefit of piperine, the doses were 2g of curcumin and 20mg of piperine.

Like active compounds in any plant, turmeric contains variable amounts of curcumin, being somewhere between 2 and 10%. This means that a dose of 2g of curcumin would require at least 20g of turmeric and as high as 100g (too much!). One teaspoon of turmeric is about 2g and provides 200mg of curcumin at best.

Piperine can be obtained as a supplement called bioperine, or more simply as ground black pepper. One writer suggested that two shakes of pepper would be 10mg, so 20mg would need four shakes.

23. GARLIC AND ITS FAMILY RESEARCH NOTES

Animal Studies (examples)

1. In rats, garlic powder prevented precancerous changes in breast cells[17].
2. In a mouse experiment, DADS from garlic reduced one type of lung cancer, but increased another[18].
3. Rats given garlic oil produced more lymphocytes (white blood cells), which make cytokines (chemical messengers) against cancer cells[19].
4. Quercetin (in onions and garlic) has anticancer activity against cancer cell lines and in rodent studies[20].

Human Population Studies

1. Medline review (1966 to 1998) of epidemiologic studies (case control and cohort control) found that a higher intake of garlic in a population resulted in a lower incidence of cancer of the stomach and large bowel. This applied to natural garlic, whereas garlic supplements did not reduce cancer risk[21].

   Examples from the Medline Review

   i You (China) found that people who ate up to 1.5kg of garlic per year (4.5g/d) had 20% less stomach cancers. If they ate more than 1.5kg/year, the risk was reduced by 30%[22].

   ii LeMarchand (Hawai) found that 2g of garlic/day was associated with a 20% reduction in risk of colorectal cancer in women but produced less benefit in men[23].

2. Prospective cohort study - followed 100,000 people who developed 1000 cancers. Garlic eaters had less bowel cancers, but only in women, not in men. Supplements were unhelpful[24].
3. A meta-analysis also showed risk reduction of stomach cancers (nearly half as many) and large bowel cancers (two-thirds) in those who ate four cloves of garlic per week compared to those who had only one or less[25]. These results are amazing, but were questioned because the studies were all a bit different. Variation in study design makes a meta-analysis less valid than if the studies had been more similar in the way they were carried out.
4. A study from Italy and Switzerland of 25,000 cancer cases with matched controls found reduction rates of 10-80% depending on the type of cancer. Onions had their greatest effect against cancer of the colon, larynx and ovary, while garlic was best against bowel and kidney cancer. Breast cancer was reduced 25% by onions, but considered not to be statistically significant[13].
5. Iowa study – 35,000 women. Those who ate one clove of garlic per week had colorectal cancer reduced by 31% compared to those who rarely ate any[14].
6. San Francisco study showed pancreatic cancer was reduced by 50% in garlic eaters[26].
7. French paper reported that garlic decreased the incidence of breast cancer[27].

How Much?

The dose of garlic needed to produce an anticancer effect, based on the studies above, has been stated as 4-5 cloves per week, or 2-4g per day. Cloves vary quite a lot and weigh from 2 to 5g, so five cloves a week is at least 10g, which corresponds to about 2g/d.

According to the WHO[28],

1 fresh clove = 2 – 5g
= 0.4 – 1.2g of garlic powder
= 2 – 5mg of garlic oil or Allium equivalent
= 300 – 1000mg of garlic extract

24. GREEN TEA RESEARCH NOTES

Human Studies

1. Nakachi, Breast cancer, in Japanese Journal of Cancer Research, 1998[27]

   472 Japanese women with breast cancer. Looked at green tea consumption prior to diagnosis and effects on prognosis. Those who drank more green tea had a lower number of involved axillary lymph nodes and after seven years of follow-up, had about half the recurrence rate (adjusted).

5 or more cups/d	17% had recurrences
less than 5 cups/d	24% had recurrences

   only applied to stage 1 and 2 disease, but no difference for stage 3

2. Kumar (type of tea not specified), in Cancer Epidemiol Biomarkers Prev, 2009[28]

   Case control study of 5082 women with breast cancer and 4501 controls.

   No overall difference in cancer risk, but a 37% reduced risk in women under 50 years of age, seen in those who had 3 or more cups of tea (black or green), compared to none.

   Black tea benefit may be due to theaflavins.

   (But perhaps the benefit would have been clearer if green tea drinkers were identified).

3. Bettuzzi, Prostate cancer, in Cancer Research, 2006[29]

   Double blind placebo-controlled, 30 in each arm.

   Biopsy-proven high grade intra-epithelial neoplasia (known to become invasive in 30% at 1 year).

Placebo - 9/30 became invasive
GTC - 1/30 became invasive
(GTC is a green tea extract of catechins, with EGCG making up >50%).

Follow up at 2 years - 2 more cancers in placebo arm, 1 more in GTC arm.

Overall, progression reduced by 80%.

4. Wu, Asian women in USA with breast cancer, in International Journal of Cancer, 2003[30]

Case control study with 501 cancer patients and 594 controls.

Compared regular green tea drinkers with those who had it <once/mth.

1 drink /d reduced breast cancer risk by 29%.

>86ml / d reduced risk by 47% (adjusted).

5. Ogunleye, Meta-analysis of breast cancer, in Breast Cancer Res Treat, 2010[31]

5617 cases

Recurrence (2 studies) - >3 cups/d reduced recurrence by 37%.

Incidence (5 studies) - case control studies showed reduction of 29% but cohort studies did not show any difference.

6. Inoue, Breast cancer recurrence study, in Cancer Letters, 2001[32]

1160 breast cancer cases.

Overall recurrence of 12%.

>3 cups/d - recurrence reduced by 31% overall.

for stage 1 - recurrence reduced by 57%, no effect on stage 3.

7. Sun, Gastric and oesophageal cancer, in Carcinogenesis, 2002[33]

Cohort of 18,244 men

Found 190 stomach cancers, 42 oesophageal cancers.

Compared them to 772 matched controls from the group.

Used urinary EGC (a green tea catechin) as a marker of green tea consumption.

EGC present in urine - reduced gastric cancers by 48%, oesophageal cancers by 42%.

Reviewed 12 other studies - 7 showed green tea to be protective, 4 not protective, 1 worse.

8. Nechuta, Digestive system cancers, in American Journal of Clinical Nutrition, 2012[34]

   >69,000 women from Shanghai Women's Study

   1255 of them developed gastro-intestinal cancers (all types) over 11 year period.

   >3 cups/wk (for at least 6 months) - 14% cancer reduction.

   The effect was greater if more tea or for longer - 3 cups/d had 21% reduction but these women also exercised more, and were better paid.

Other Studies

- Leukoplakia - green tea increased regression rate[35].
- Liver cancer patients with Hepatitis C and aflatoxin exposure - cancer marker reduced by green tea[36].
- Cancer of cervix, relative risk (RR) of cancer was 0.55 in patients with precancerous change[37].
- Bladder cancer meta-analysis - RR 0.81[38]
- Colorectal cancer meta-analysis - RR 0.95 (weak benefit)[39]

Mechanisms of Action Of Green Tea[1,40-46]

- Arrests the cell cycle and promotes apoptosis.
- Inhibits Ras/MAPK pathway (Ras mutations and activation produce cell growth signals).
- Inhibits PI3kinase/Akt "pro-survival signalling pathway".
- Inhibits **tyrosine kinase** (see Footnote), to block the IGF1 pathway.
- Inhibits transcription factors which are needed for expression of DNA e.g. **nuclear factor kappaB (NFkB)**, activator protein1 (AP1). NFkappaB is a late product of a signalling pathway. It is able to enter the nucleus and transcribe many genes, including genes that suppress apoptosis or induce proliferation.
- Prevents invasion and metastases - blocks urokinase plasminogen activator (uPA), matrix metalloproteases, and hyaluronidase.
- Inhibits COX 2 expression (inflammation).
- Inhibits telomerase. **Telomerase** maintains telomere nuclear end caps and allows an unlimited number of cell divisions. Normal cells lose ends of DNA with each division, eventually leading to senescence (ageing and loss of regeneration). Telomerase is

increased in many cancers, contributing to their "immortal" status.
- Stabilizes p53 (for apoptosis).
- Blocks angiogenesis – blocks VEGF and IL8 (proangiogenic cytokine).
- Inhibits proteosomes. These are needed for various signalling pathways, in releasing active proteins to keep the cascade rolling.
- Inhibits expression of androgen receptors (may have a role in androgen sensitive prostate cancer).
- Promotes gap junctional cell communication - blocks tumour growth by sealing receptors.
- Binds carcinogens.
- Antioxidant - free radical scavenging protects against DNA damage.
- Protects against UVB damage when applied topically.
- Activates detoxifying enzymes, including glutathione-s-transferase.

Additionally, green tea:
- Improves function of intestinal flora.
- Helps reduce body weight.
- Improves bone density and reduces hip fracture rate, important in some breast cancer patients[47,48].

Footnote on **tyrosine kinase**: A cell membrane receptor is part of a complex structure, with the receptor being on the outer surface of the cell. This part is stimulated by a specific substance (such as a growth factor) which comes into contact with the cell. The receptor is connected to a section that projects through the cell membrane to the inside of the cell. This inner part has an enzyme called tyrosine kinase which is activated when the receptor is stimulated. Tyrosine kinase then triggers changes in many internal cell chemicals, which is the beginning of a cascade (signalling pathway) leading to genes being expressed (e.g. causing growth). Also see figure in "Signalling pathways", p.121.

25. FLAXSEEDS RESEARCH NOTES

OMEGA 3 OILS

Types of Oil

As mentioned, the main players on a rather complex stage are:

Omega 3, two broad sources:

1. Fatty fish (e.g. salmon, sardines) or krill
   - provides EPA (eicosapentaenoic acid) and DHA (docosa-hexaenoic acid).
2. Vegetables, especially flaxseed (also called linseed) and walnuts
   - provide ALA (alpha-linolenic acid)
   which can be converted into EPA and DHA, after ingestion.

Omega 6, key members:

1. Linoleic oil (LA) is the main Omega 6 oil and dominates the available vegetable oils, particularly sunflower, safflower, corn, soy and canola oils.
2. Arachidonic acid is Omega 6 and pro-inflammatory. It is derived from LA, and in meat.
3. CLA (conjugated linoleic acid) is found in meat from grass-fed cows (less if grain fed)[10]. Despite being an Omega 6, it may protect against cancer[11].
4. GLA (gamma-linolenic acid) comes from evening primrose oil, black currant seed oil and borage oil. Although an Omega 6 oil, it is useful in promoting conversion of ALA to DHA/EPA.

Olive oil is mainly Omega 9.

Fish versus Flax[12-17]

There is some debate over whether we should obtain Omega 3 from plants (ALA) or fish (DHA, EPA).

This is quite complicated and involves whether ALA can be readily converted to DHA and EPA, which then lead on to the beneficial anti-inflammatory cytokines (cell messengers). Otherwise, they go down the path to the inflammatory ones via arachidonic acid. The conversion process, requiring desaturase enzymes, can be inhibited by high insulin levels (obesity, diabetes, carbohydrate loading), alcohol, transfats, viral infections, ageing, and even by the fatty acids themselves. Genetic variation also plays a role, with conversion being poor in certain ethnic groups such as North American natives, Orientals, Welsh-Irish, and Norwegians. On the other hand, conversion improves with GLA supplementation.

For those focusing on plant sources of Omega 3 (ALA from flaxseeds), conversion to DHA and EPA can be enhanced by reducing the intake of Omega 6 and transfats, avoiding obesity, and taking a GLA supplement. It is argued that ALA (from plants) is important in its own right and various body tissues will make the conversion according to their needs.

Marine sources are already in the form of DHA and EPA, not requiring further conversion, but may be contaminated with mercury, heavy metals, dioxins, PCBs, pesticides and other pollutants. Fish with high mercury levels include shark, swordfish, and king mackerel. These are the large ones that have lived long enough to accumulate toxins. Fish meals should be limited to two per week. A supplement should be safer, but may still be contaminated. Krill is less likely to have accumulated toxins because they are small organisms. Krill oil also has a beneficial phospholipid component which may aid incorporation into cell membranes.

Flaxseeds, as well as being the key vegetable source of Omega 3s, have the added anticancer effects of lignans and fibre.

Given the diversity of opinion, it would seem wise to seek Omega 3 oils from both plant and marine sources. For example, eat flaxseeds, and take a reputable fish oil supplement (or eat more sardines and salmon).

Animal Research

Omega 3 supplements inhibit breast cancer cells in cell cultures and in mice cancer grafts[18].

In rats, canola oil decreased colon cancer incidence compared to corn oil (which is mainly Omega 6), and this was associated with lower COX-2 expression (marker of inflammation) in colon samples[19].

Rats given flaxseed meal (compared to corn) were shown to have vastly lower incidence, number and size of colon tumours. This was seen to be related to high Omega 6 levels in blood and tissue for corn, and high Omega 3 for flaxseed[20].

In a mouse model with human breast cancer cells, a fish oil diet prevented bone metastases. DHA/EPA attenuates cancer cell migration and invasion. They inhibit CD44 protein expression, which has a role in the generation of cancer stem cells[21].

Mice given walnuts developed breast cancer at less than half the rate[22].

Human Studies: Breast and Prostate Cancer

In the VITAL study cohort of 35,000 postmenopausal women, those who used fish oil at the time of the survey had a rate of breast cancer 32% less than the non-users[23].

Omega 3s lowered the risk of breast and prostate cancer via an effect on intracellular adhesion molecules (ICAM) in a French study which assessed 408 cancer patients and 760 controls[24].

Another French study looked at 241 breast cancer patients and 88 with benign breast disease. Those with cancer had a higher Omega 6: Omega 3 ratio in biopsies of their adipose tissue[25].

In a case control study of prostate cancer, a high Omega 6: Omega 3 ratio increased the risk of high grade cancer (but no difference for low grade prostate cancer)[26]. It should be mentioned that another study suggested the opposite, with an increased risk of prostate cancer in men with high DHA (Omega 3) levels[27]. However, the source of DHA was unknown, the 6:3 ratio was unknown, and there were other gaps in the study[28].

Mechanisms of Action of Omega 3 Oils

- Mediterranean diets (generally high in fish and olive oil) are not all the same, and many mechanisms are recognized[29,30].

- Chronic inflammation is increasingly being recognized as a cause of cancer, and Omega 3 oils, being anti-inflammatory, can play a role against it in this respect. (see p.122)
- Omega 3s inhibit eicosanoid production (from Omega 6), and suppress pro-inflammatory COX-2, IL-1 and IL-6 gene expression[30].
- Metabolites of arachidonic acid (Omega 6) inhibit apoptosis and stimulate proliferation by up-regulating cyclin D1 expression. Omega 3 metabolites do the opposite by down-regulating cyclin D1[31].
- Arachidonic acid and DHA have opposite roles in protein binding in gliomas (brain tumours), favouring or blocking cell migration, respectively[32].
- Omega 3s have a role in reverting (cancerous) glycolytic metabolism to (healthy) oxidative metabolism which enhances sensitivity to apoptosis. Cancer cells have resistance to apoptosis, but this can be reversed by this kind of "metabolic reprogramming"[33].
- Omega 3s block angiogenesis[34].
- Olive oil contains polyphenols (including secoiridoids, lignans) which inhibit HER2 tyrosine kinase and degrade HER2 protein. This works against breast cancer synergistically with the drug Herceptin (trastuzamab). However, the levels obtained in the lab were probably above those achievable in vivo (an actual living human)[35].
- Omega 3s lower the levels of circulating soluble adhesion molecules involved in inflammation and carcinogenesis[24].
- GLA becomes incorporated into cell membranes and prevents the genetic influences of NFkappaB[36].

LIGNANS

Research

There are plenty of animal studies showing that a lignan-rich diet reduces a number of cancer types, including breast and melanoma. It slows the growth of the main (primary) tumour and also lowers the number of metastases.

For humans, consider the evidence below:

Breast cancer

A small randomized trial focused on women having surgery for breast cancer, with the cancer tissue being removed and analysed. In the ones who were given flaxseed muffins leading up to surgery, the tumour markers of proliferation and aggression were reduced compared to those who had muffins without flaxseed[37].

Lignans have been shown to decrease the risk of getting breast cancer in the first place, but equally impressively, reduce the risk of death after diagnosis, too. 1140 breast cancer patients had their blood levels of enterolactone (from lignans) measured and were followed for six years, during which time many of them died from the disease. The risk of dying was much lower in the ones with highest levels of enterolactone. In fact, they were 40% less likely to die. The protection was even greater for the oestrogen-receptor negative cancers. The ER positive ones had some protection, but not to a statistically significant level[38,39].

Bowel cancer

A dietary questionnaire was given to over a thousand patients who had colorectal cancer, and compared to controls. Lignan intake was associated with a reduced cancer risk of 37%[40]. Colorectal adenomas (precancerous polyps) are less likely to occur in people who have high levels of enterodiol (from lignans) in their blood[41].

Prostate cancer

Case control studies from Sweden[42], Scotland[43] and New York[44] all looked at blood levels of enterolactones (from lignans) and found a reduced risk of prostate cancer in those with the highest levels, with the reduction ranging from 34% to 82%.

Mechanisms of Action of Lignans

Lignan products (enterolactone, enterodiol) block growth receptors like EGF (endothelial growth factor), HER2 (human epidermal growth factor), and IGF-1 (insulin-like growth factor)[45].

They block angiogenesis via VEGF (vascular endothelial growth factor)[46].

As phyto-oestrogens, they can block oestrogen receptors. They also favour the enzymes that convert oestrogen to its less dangerous form, and are involved in testosterone metabolism[47].

Enterolactone blocks tyrosine kinase (a growth signaller in both breast and prostate cancer)[48,49], and promotes apoptosis.

26. MUSHROOMS RESEARCH NOTES

Studies

1. Adjuvant PSK (Japan)[14] (PSK is polysaccharide peptide K, from Coriolus mushroom)

	Chemo alone	Chemo **plus PSK**
After surgery for Stomach cancer		
No recurrence at 5 yrs	60%	73%
After surgery for Colorectal cancer		
No recurrence at 5yrs (Stage 2 + 3)	59%	73%
No recurrence at 5yrs (Stage 3)	32%	60%

2. Adjuvant Lentinan (Japan)[15]

   Lentinan is an extract from Shiitake mushrooms. Used with chemo, it improved survival in stomach and colorectal cancers compared to chemo alone. When used alone, Lentinan was ineffective against prostate cancer.

3. Mushroom consumption

   Case control studies – five published papers of note, all cases from China, Japan or Korea.

Author	Number of cases/ controls	Cancer type	Variable	Result
Zhang et al[16]	1009/1009	Breast (BC)	>10g fresh	64% decrease in BC
			4-10g fresh	47% decrease in BC
			Plus Green Tea	89% decrease in BC
(significant for both pre- and post-menopausal women)				
Hong et al[4]	362/362	Breast	15g vs 0g	1/6th incidence of BC
(but only statistically significant for postmenopausal women)				
Shin et al[17]	358/360	Breast	>11g vs <3g	1/3 incidence of BC
(but only statistically significant for premenopausal women)				
Lee et al[18]	189/189	Breast		"Mushrooms decreased breast cancer risk"
Hara et al[19]	147/287	GIT		"Mushrooms decreased stomach cancer risk"

Statistical significance was not reached for all groups. The conflicting results between pre- and post-menopausal women may reflect smallish numbers, and larger numbers may have clarified it.

Mechanisms of Action of Mushrooms[1,10,20,21]

1. Immune system

Beta-glucans are large "polysaccharide" molecules, contained in mushrooms. There are many structural differences, so not all beta-glucans have anticancer effects. Some have sugar or protein side-arms and various branching shapes. Their size and structural variability provides the potential to act on cells, to regulate cell-to-cell interactions.

Our immune cells actually carry surface receptors for beta-glucans. This allows identification of these molecules by our immune system as "non-self", triggering the activation of lymphocytes, macrophages, dendritic cells, and natural killer (NK) cells. These cells then act against cancer cells, both at the primary site and those "in-transit" within blood vessels and lymphatics, thus preventing metastases. Beta-glucans stimulate production of cytokines (chemicals that further attract and activate more immune cells) such as interleukins, tumour necrosis factor and interferon, all of which play an anticancer role[22]. Many experiments have shown that mushroom extracts have these effects on the immune system.

2. Aromatase inhibition

   Pharmaceutical aromatase inhibitors work by blocking oestrogen production and are used against oestrogen-positive breast cancer in standard medical practice. They are extremely effective. Several mushrooms, including Button, Shiitake, Portobello, Crimius, and Baby Button, are able to suppress aromatase. It does not mean that they can replace prescribed aromatase inhibitors.

3. Enhancement of chemotherapy

   As noted in the clinical trials above, patients can survive longer when given mushroom extracts alongside chemotherapy. This is also seen in the lab where, for example, Maitake mushroom extract enhances cisplatin. Lion's mane mushroom enhances doxorubicin. The Japanese trials also showed significant reduction in many side effects of chemo[7], presumably by countering the immune suppression caused by chemo.

   Grifron-D (GD) from Grifola (Maitake) inactivates glyoxalase 1, which would otherwise metabolize chemotherapy agents. This means that GD increases their availability.

4. Direct effects on cancer cells

   Reishi mushrooms cause apoptosis via mitochondrial dysfunction and cell cycle arrest. They contain ganoderic acid, which inhibits invasion and metastasis. Invasion and migration are also blocked by Ganoderma[6] and by PSK, which prevents tumour cell production of proteinases (enzymes that break down host tissues, allowing tumour invasion).

   Maitake mushrooms contain S-GAP-P, a sulphated polysaccharide, which induces apoptosis (cell suicide). Apoptosis is also promoted by cordycepin (from Cordyceps), and by Winter mushroom which is effective against both oestrogen-receptor negative and ER positive breast cancer cells.

5. Other anticancer mechanisms

As well as acting on the immune system, beta-glucans block angiogenesis by working against proangiogenic factors like VEGF, COX2 and 5LOX.

Effect on stem cells: In prostate cancer, PSP in Coriolus (Turkey tail) mushroom targets cancer stem cells[23]. Stem cells are thought to evade chemotherapy and hence, can be responsible for cancer recurrence. In mice, PSP supplement resulted in complete prevention of prostate cancer, whereas the untreated mice all developed the cancer. However, the dose required was more than can be achieved by dietary supplements. Cordlan in Cordyceps mushrooms has a beneficial effect on stem cells by aiding their maturation.

Mushrooms also contain anticancer compounds discussed elsewhere, including selenium, antioxidants and fibre. Fibre absorbs potential carcinogens while in the bowel, hastening their elimination and reducing the risk of colorectal cancer.

27. RESVERATROL, GRAPES, AND RED WINE RESEARCH NOTES

Resveratrol Content (in descending order)[1,3,16,17]

Red wine	0.2 – 8 mg/l (on average less than 1mg per glass)
Red grapes	1mg per cup (160g)
Grape juice	0.5 mg/l
Blueberries	<10% of grape content
Peanuts	0.08 mg/ounce (= 15 peanuts), x 5 if sprouted

Grape Types, Regions and Resveratrol Levels[18-20]

The grape types with the most resveratrol include Malbec and Pinot Noir. Grapes from warm climates will have less than those from cool climates, because the warm grape-growing regions are usually drier so there is less fungal growth, and fungus stimulates resveratrol production. Also north of the equator is better. Wines

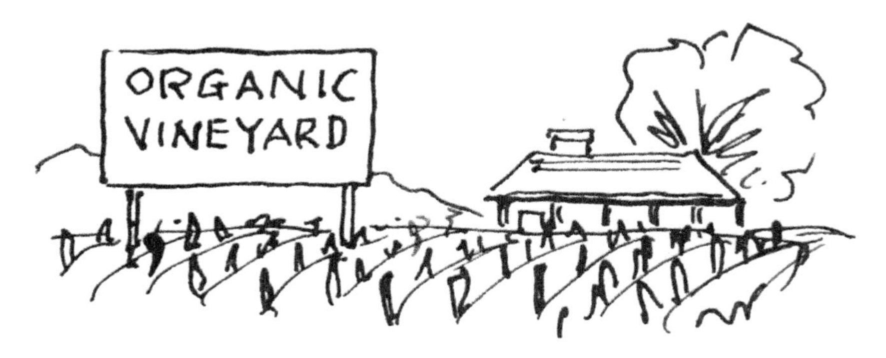

from Canada, Northern USA, and Germany contain more than those from Australia, South Africa and Italy. However, grapes cultured in the zone of the equator also contain resveratrol in high concentration, because of higher ultraviolet radiation.

The levels in a single grape can change from week to week depending on conditions. One grower in Spain claims to have learned how to somehow stress the grapes before harvesting, resulting in a very high resveratrol level. In contrast, "resveratrol-enhanced wine" has resveratrol artificially added later. Another successful way of increasing resveratrol in grapes is to subject them to UV radiation after harvesting[21].

Wines made from Muscadine grapes can have up to eight times more resveratrol than average, but even these have large variations. Muscadine grapes have tough thick skins which range from bronze to dark purple to black in colour, and are often used for port, or sweet (dessert) wine. They also contain catechins, ellagic acid and other polyphenols.

Concord grapes are recommended for the "Brandt Grape Cure" for cancer, but I'm not sure why they would be better than other red grapes.

Bioavailability[22-25]

Having seen the incredible array of anticancer effects of resveratrol in the laboratory, it is disappointing to discover that there are some doubts about whether a dietary source would be effective. Initial absorption from the bowel is excellent, but it is rapidly metabolized by the liver, so that the amount of resveratrol in the blood is reduced to almost nil. This does not affect resveratrol reaching the cells that line the gastrointestinal tract (mouth, oesophagus, bowel) which take it up quickly by direct contact. In humans, resveratrol does reach colon cancer tissue in useful quantities after oral ingestion[26]. Indeed, the benefits in lab animals have been seen primarily against colon cancer.

To prevent cancers in other internal organs, we would expect that a certain blood level is required. The liver modifies resveratrol by adding sulphate or glucuronide to it (conjugation). These metabolites are certainly detectable in the blood, but have not been recognized as having anticancer actions, given that the lab work has focused on resveratrol itself. The "conjugation/deconjugation" concept is that these metabolites enter the cells and, once inside, the sulphate or glucuronide is removed, leaving resveratrol inside the cell to do its good work. This would mean that all organs could benefit. The glucuronidase or sulphatase enzymes required for this conversion have been reported as being higher in some target tissues, such as those affected by inflammation or malignancy[27].

Blood levels may be better if resveratrol is taken with a meal. Quercetin probably does not help, despite some claims.

Related to resveratrol is a phytochemical called pterostilbene (which is another name for methylresveratrol). This is present in grapes and blueberries and also has anticancer activity. It seems to have better bioavailability. Unlike resveratrol, it survives several passes through the liver before being metabolized. It is promoted as better by some writers, but research is limited.

28. SELENIUM RESEARCH NOTES

Mechanisms of Action

Selenium:

1. Is needed for synthesis of selenoproteins, such as glutathione peroxidase (an antioxidant) and glutathione transferase, which deactivates environmental carcinogens.
2. Induces apoptosis. If a malignant cell is halted partway through splitting to become two malignant cells ("cell cycle arrest"), and its mutated DNA cannot be repaired, it can then be pushed into apoptosis. It self destructs and is removed. Selenium is able to arrest the cell cycle to achieve this[20]. In addition, it induces apoptosis by deactivating protein kinase C (which has a role in cell survival)[21].
3. Improves the immune system. Selenium doubles the cancer-killing ability of cytotoxic lymphocytes (CTLs) and natural killer cells[22]. This is partly attributed to selenium increasing the IL-2 receptors on the lymphocytes, thus activating them[23]. In animals, selenium restores loss of CTL ability caused by advancing age. Nursing home residents given selenium have an enhanced lymphocyte response to foreign antigens[24].

The antioxidant function of selenoproteins is important against cancer, but in fact, a normal diet will usually provide enough selenium to keep the selenoproteins supplied. If a higher intake of selenium is achieved, the excess (left over after manufacture of selenoproteins) is then available for its apoptotic effect, which may be more important against cancer.

Zinc Problem

Drake takes a strong position against zinc, claiming that it blocks the apoptotic effect of selenium by inhibiting the enzyme endonuclease, which chops up cancer cell DNA. This could explain why the selenium in the fourth Chinese study[10] was ineffective, and perhaps why the SUVIMAX study from France showed mixed results[25]. Experimentally, zinc allows proliferation of prostate cancer cells by enhancing telomerase activity. Telomerase enables cells to divide virtually forever, endowing cancer cells with immortality. Zinc may also interfere with absorption of selenium.

However, others are in favour of zinc as an anticancer agent. Perhaps a middle-of-the-road approach would be to not take selenium and zinc together, even though they often co-exist in commercial multivitamins. Zinc supplements will usually be unnecessary due to its presence in many food sources such as seafood, meat, seeds, nuts and beans.

Brazil Nuts versus Supplements of Selenomethionine (SM)

A New Zealand paper compared consumption of Brazil nuts to a selenium supplement as selenomethionine(SM), and found that both groups achieved an increase in plasma levels of selenium. However, those who took the nuts had a higher whole blood level and a higher level of glutathione peroxidase activity, suggesting that the selenium from the nuts was more bioavailable[12]. The main form of selenium in Brazil nuts is SM, but at least 20% is in other forms, implying that it is these other forms that made the difference, as with Clark's study which used high selenium yeast.

The key anticancer molecule is methylselenol. The biochemical pathways are depicted in the diagram on the next page. MSC is directly converted to methylselenol. In contrast, SM can be directed to general body proteins in place of sulfur (top left of diagram) or to selenoproteins (top right). The SM which enters (and becomes stored in) general body proteins is not functioning in any way against cancer, but will give false reassurance that a person's selenium levels are good when measured in skin, nails or hair. The SM which is converted to specific selenoproteins (such as glutathione peroxidase) will serve an anticancer purpose as an antioxidant. However, not much SM goes through the key methylselenol pathway. In comparison, it makes sense that MSC (e.g. from high selenium garlic) will be more

Figure: Metabolic pathway of dietary selenium (simplified) [1,26,27]

This figure shows two dietary forms or supplements, SM and MSC. It illustrates how MSC is more directly converted to methylselenol for anticancer effects, compared to SM which may also lead to the formation of methylselenol, but is readily diverted to protein production, instead.

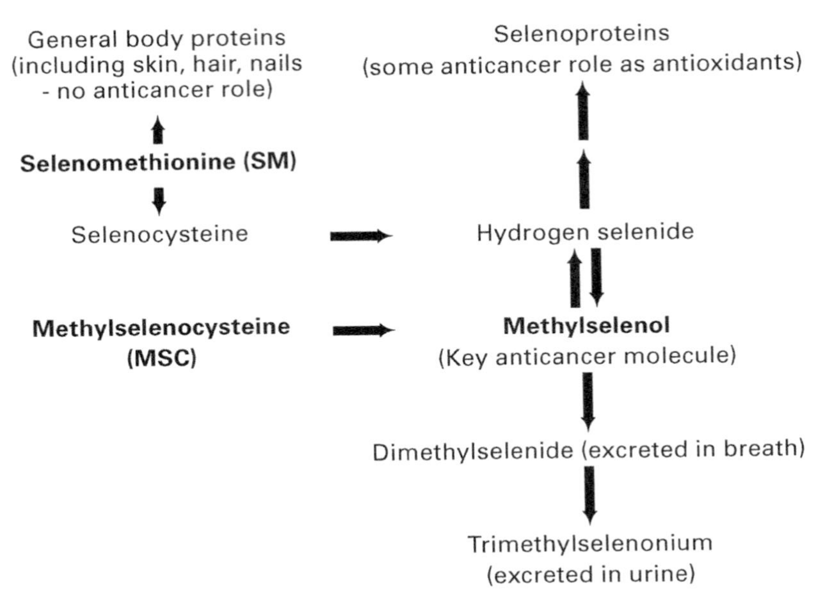

effective than SM because it leads to formation of methylselenol to a much greater degree. MSC is also converted to selenoproteins, but is not diverted to general body proteins.

Dimethylselenide is exhaled and contributes to the characteristic garlic breath. This occurs when the amount exceeds what can be excreted in the urine as trimethylselenonium. The point is that these metabolic steps continually remove selenium, which means that to maintain useful levels of methylselenol, a regular intake of selenium is required.

Recommended Dose

The effective and safe doses outlined in Chapter 9 refer to the selenium content. For example methylselenocysteine (MSC) is about 43% selenium by weight, meaning 100mcg of MSC would contain 43mcg of selenium. Supplement labelling usually allows for this, and states the amount of actual selenium.

29. CARROTS, CAROTENE AND COLOUR RESEARCH NOTES

How Do Carotenoids Work Against Cancer?

Firstly, they have an antioxidant and free radical scavenging effect (prevents cell damage).

Healthy volunteers took either carotene supplements or carrots or placebos, and then had blood samples taken. White blood cells in the sample were then deliberately damaged with hydrogen peroxide. Blood from the volunteers who took carotene or carrots showed accelerated repair of DNA damage, implying that carrot eaters may be protected from this form of cancer initiation[14].

Secondly, there is an antiproliferative action (prevents cancer cell growth).

This is probably due to the vitamin A, which has different forms. Alpha- and beta-carotenes are vitamin A precursors (they are converted to vitamin A).

The retinal form of vitamin A is important in vision. Retinol is the transport and storage form. The retinoic acid form regulates cell differentiation and growth. It can cause cancer cells to undergo apoptosis (self destruction) or differentiation (i.e. to revert to normal behaviour)[15,16]. We don't have to kill cancer cells if we can change them. Men with low levels of vitamin A have long been known to have worse prostate cancers[17]. Beta-carotene can also enhance cell-mediated immunity, even after less than a month of supplements[18].

Lycopene and retinoic acid from tomatoes and carrots block insulin-like growth factor (IGF)[19]. IGF promotes cancer. Lycopene also inhibits angiogenesis[20].

Carotenoids from diet have been shown to enter the skin and protect from UV radiation[21].

Falcarinol is a more recently identified phytochemical in carrots, celery and parsley. It is a natural pesticide, protecting carrots from fungal disease. In the lab it has some anticancer effects[22]. These are largely lost when the carrots are cooked[23].

Problems with Supplements

100g of raw carrots (one and a half carrots, or half a cup) provides 17000 units of vitamin A which is plenty (three times the recommended allowance). Low levels appear to be the danger (especially for prostate cancer), and it seems that we only need to aim for normal levels, not super high ones. Too much vitamin A is toxic, but in practice this is only caused by supplements or animal sources such as liver. Plant sources are not a problem because the body won't convert excess dietary carotenes to vitamin A. On this point, although high dietary beta-carotene reduces lung cancer[24], beta-carotene supplements were shown to increase the risk in smokers[25]. Stick with natural food sources. In a review of beta-carotenes as supplements, no reduction in cancer risk was seen[26]. Over and again, for most things, we see that food is superior to a tablet.

30. PROBIOTICS RESEARCH NOTES

Bladder Cancer

Probiotics containing Lactobacillus casei have been shown to prevent the recurrence of bladder cancer[6].

In a study by Hayatsu[7], subjects were given fried ground beef to eat. Those who were also given Lactobacillus were found to have less heterocyclic amines in their urine and faeces, indicating that the probiotics were negating the carcinogenic toxins from the fried meat.

Colorectal Cancer

In rats, probiotics prevent colorectal cancer, and in human colon cancer cell lines, lactic acid bacilli (LAB) cause inhibition of growth[8].

In a study by Ishikara[9], 4000 patients with a history of colorectal cancer were followed for four years and were supplemented with either wheat bran, probiotics, neither, or both. There was no difference in the number who developed polyps, but in those who received the probiotics, the polyps appeared more slowly.

SYNCAN[10]: This European study looked at supplementation with probiotics and prebiotics for 12 weeks in patients after treatment of bowel polyps or bowel cancer. The bowel lining was biopsied at the start and finish. Those who received the supplements had 60% less DNA damage, less cell proliferation, and less carcinogens in their faeces.

Epidemiology: At least three studies have shown that greater consumption of yoghurt was associated with a lower rate of colorectal cancer[11-13].

Breast Cancer

Consumption of fermented dairy products is linked to reduced breast cancer risk[14]. In one study, 133 breast cancer patients were compared to 289 controls. The cancer group had a significantly lower consumption of fermented milk products such as yoghurt and buttermilk[15].

Anticancer mechanisms of beneficial bacteria in the gut lumen[16-21]

They:

- Detoxify aflatoxin which promotes liver cancer.
- Suppress bad bacteria and putrefactive organisms like yeasts.

  They do this by competing with them for nutrients, or directly consuming them, thus preventing their production of carcinogens.

- Inhibit the beta-glucuronidase enzyme produced by harmful bacteria.

  Glucuronidase acts on glucuronides in the bile to produce aglycones, which are carcinogenic. Glucuronidases prevent detoxification of oestrogen (from oestradiol to oestriol). The reduction in such enzymes from probiotics is temporary, with levels rising again within 30 days of ceasing the supplement. Also, these unfavourable enzyme levels are higher in omnivores eating a Western diet than in vegetarians. The levels cannot simply be lowered by reducing meat or adding fibre, but a reduction can be achieved with probiotics.

- Deconjugate bile acids.

  Bile acids increase as a result of a high fat diet. They are reabsorbed from the bowel and then re-excreted by the liver (enterohepatic circulation), but eventually progress to the colon where their breakdown products are toxic to colonic epithelium. Beneficial bacteria reduce the levels of bile acids.

- Improve general immunity.

  This is by enhancing Natural Killer cells, and increasing levels of immunoglobulins and cytokines (including interferon, IL-1, TNFalpha). This may be how probiotics reduce the risk of other cancers beyond the bowel. Another way is by reducing absorption of toxins that would otherwise be excreted in the urine later, raising the risk of bladder cancer.

- Increase antioxidant enzymes.

  Enzymes such as glutathione-S-transferase protect cells from oxidative DNA damage.

- Produce butyrate.

  Butyrate is a short-chain fatty acid produced by the action of bacteria on fibre. It stabilizes DNA during replication to minimize DNA damage and malignant transformation of colon lining cells. In colon cancer cell lines, butyrate causes apoptosis and blocks metastases. Butyrate (and proprionate) inhibit histone deacetylase. This allows the acetylation process in colon cancer cells to occur, activating the genes which control the cell cycle, to prevent cancer cell reproduction.

- Form CLA (conjugated linoleic acid), a fatty acid which is anti-inflammatory and inhibits cancer.
- Release cancer-preventive vitamins such as B12, folate and biotin from food.
- Modulate the anticancer immune effects of some chemotherapy agents[22].

Prebiotics

The key molecules contained in prebiotic foods are inulin (long chains of fructose)[19] and oligofructose (short chains). These are both a type of carbohydrate, but are also a dietary fibre because they cannot be digested. They pass through to the large bowel where they can be metabolized by beneficial bacteria, whose growth they stimulate.

Prebiotics and probiotics can be combined, and when used together are termed synbiotics.

31. IODINE RESEARCH NOTES

Continuing on from Chapter 13 which gives the first five points, here are further reasons why iodine may protect against cancer:

6. Most of the iodine in the body is taken up by the thyroid, but is also present in other tissues, including the breast. Uptake by breast tissue is particularly marked when pregnant or lactating, in order to pass on iodine to the baby. We know that pregnancy protects against breast cancer. This has been partly attributed to the fact that pregnancy interrupts the repeated oestrogen stimulation that comes with normal menstrual cycles. However, it should be considered that the higher concentrations of iodine in the breast over this period may be a key factor in eliminating cancer precursor cells[5], and thus preventing the appearance of breast cancer at a later date.

In non-lactating women, the low level of iodine intake from a western diet is insufficient to reach the breast because it will all go to the thyroid. A much higher intake is needed to saturate the thyroid's requirement in order for the surplus to reach the other tissues.

7. In tissues that contain peroxidase enzymes such as the thyroid and breast, iodine binds with fats to form iodolipids (including iodolactones) which inhibit cell proliferation[15] and promote apoptosis[16]. Iodolactones (iodine bound to arachidonic acid) inhibit epidermal growth factor (EGF) receptors and mediate apoptosis. This certainly has a role in preventing thyroid enlargement (goitre), and may also control the proliferation of breast tissue.

8. Iodine has an antioxidant effect which protects against cancer. Electrons are transferred from iodine to the oxygen on hydrogen peroxidase, which protects breast tissue from (lipo) peroxidation[17].
9. In rats, progesterone reduces breast cancers, but this effect is increased when iodine is also given[18]. The tumours which had suppressed growth were found to have higher iodine content, and it is thought that progesterone increases iodine uptake by cells. It could also be that resistant tumours did not take up the iodine because their iodine transporters were mutated or damaged[19]. The lack of iodine may have allowed them to grow more.
10. Iodine deficiency appears to be a tumour promoter rather than carcinogenic of itself (first cause of the cancer). The rate of cancer formation increases when a carcinogen is accompanied by iodine deficiency. One author theorizes that iodine deficiency allows in-situ (non-invasive) lesions to appear, and that subsequent low thyroid hormone levels allow them to become invasive through loss of a connective tissue barrier[2].
11. Iodine deficiency causes an increase in thyroid stimulating hormone (TSH), as well as an increased cell responsiveness to the TSH. Iodine deficiency leads to angiogenesis (formation of new blood vessels). This is useful in increasing blood flow to a thyroid that is struggling to make enough thyroid hormone, but it can also aid tumour growth. Cancers need new blood vessels in order to progress. The mechanism here is via blood vessel growth factors such as vascular endothelial growth factor (VEGF-A)[20].

APPENDIX: USEFUL RESOURCES

Books

There are dozens of books on the subject of diet and cancer, not all of which I would necessarily recommend. Authors include medical doctors, research scientists, investigative journalists, celebrities, cancer survivors, nutritionists, and alternative therapists. If you are reading widely, reserve judgement until you are convinced that you can trust the author's credentials and competence. Even then, look for other reliable sources that agree on any particular topic.

The following are the books that originally caught my interest, and I recommend:

- "The China Study" by T Colin Campbell PhD and Thomas Campbell
  (outlines the research journey of a mainstream doctor who learned the dangers of a diet based on animal products)
- "Anticancer: A New Way of Life" by Dr David Servan-Schreiber
  (a science researcher is diagnosed with a brain tumour and discovers evidence to support lifestyle changes against cancer)
- "Foods That Fight Cancer" by Richard Belliveau PhD and Denis Gingras PhD
  (describes and illustrates categories of foods against cancer)
- "In Defence of Food" by Michael Pollan
  (not specifically about cancer, but reveals the evils of the Western diet and how to counter it)

Websites

There is so much on the internet that it easily becomes overwhelming and time-wasting. These ones seem quite good but you still need to exercise your own judgement.

- American Institute for Cancer Research - http://www.aicr.org
- Cancer Active - http://canceractive.com
- Nutrition Facts.org - http://nutritionfacts.org/topics/cancer

You will also be able to find online forums and discussion groups.

Recipes

Look for meals that are in keeping with the principles you have learned. Adapt recipes you already know to include as wide a variety of anticancer foods as possible. If you need some ideas, try these:

- "Cooking with Foods That Fight Cancer" by Richard Belliveau PhD and Denis Gingras PhD
- Physicians Committee for Responsible Medicine recipes - http://pcrm.org/health/diets/recipes
- The World's Healthiest Foods recipes - www.whfoods.org

These websites also offer to send a weekly recipe by email.

Scientific Journals

Listed below are some of the most frequently cited journals on the subject of food and cancer. They can all be found online. It is an interesting exercise to go to any of their websites and type in "Broccoli" or "Garlic" to see what a huge array of research articles have been published. Likewise, a staggering number of papers will appear if you do the same searches on PubMed (www.ncbi.nlm.nih.gov/pubmed), which accesses the Medline database of biomedical topics.

- American Journal of Clinical Nutrition
- American Journal of Epidemiology
- Anticancer Research
- British Journal of Nutrition
- Cancer Causes Control
- Cancer, Epidemiology, Biomarkers, and Prevention
- Cancer Letters

- Cancer Prevention Research
- Cancer Research
- Clinical Cancer Research
- Carcinogenesis
- International Journal of Cancer
- Journal of Agriculture and Food Chemistry
- Journal of Clinical Oncology
- Journal of Nutrition
- Nutrition and Cancer
- Nutrition Research

REFERENCES

References are given together for the corresponding chapters in Parts 1 and 2. It has been done this way to keep the relevant topical references in one place. References are mainly research and review articles published in journals, but there are also some references to websites, papers or opinions which are considered helpful and reasonably accurate.

References for Introduction

1. Campbell TC, Campbell TM. The China Study. Benbella Books, Texas. 2006
2. A national centre of excellence. Article in Surgical News (Royal Australasian College of Surgeons) April 2009;10(3):31
3. Snow D. Her life's work. Good Weekend (Sydney Morning Herald) Aug 16, 2008:29-33
4. Gawler, I. You can conquer cancer. 2012. Michelle Anderson Publishing
5. Oz, M. What I learned from my cancer scare. Time Magazine June 27, 2001:31-35
6. Beliveau R, Gingras D. Foods to Fight Cancer: Essential foods to help prevent cancer. 2007. DK Adult

References for Chapters 1 and 20: Broccoli and the crucifers

1. Fowke JH, Shu X, Dai Q, Shintani A, Conaway CC, Chung F, Cai Q, Gao Y, Zheng W. Urinary Isothiocyanate Excretion, Brassica Consumption, and Gene Polymorphisms among Women Living in Shanghai, China. Cancer Epidemiology, Biomarkers & Prevention 2003 Dec(12):1536–1539
2. Matusheski NV, Juvik JA, Jeffery EH. Heating decreases epithiospecifier protein activity and increases sulforaphane formation in broccoli. Phytochemistry. 2004 May;65(9):1273-81.
3. Song L, Thornalley PJ. Effect of storage, processing and cooking on glucosinolate content of Brassica vegetables. Food Chem Toxicol. 2007 Feb;45(2):216-24.
4. Cramer JM, Teran-Garcia M, Jeffery EH. Enhancing sulforaphane absorption and excretion in healthy men through the combined consumption of

fresh broccoli sprouts and a glucoraphanin-rich powder. British Journal of Nutrition 2012;107:1333–1338

5. Force LE, O'Hare TJ, Wong LS, Irving DE. Impact of cold storage on glucosinolate levels in seed-sprouts of broccoli, rocket, white radish and kohlrabi. Postharvest Biology and Technology, 2007;44 (2):175-178.
6. Fahey JW, Zhang Y, Talalay P. Broccoli sprouts: An exceptionally rich source of inducers of enzymes that protect against chemical carcinogens. Proc. Natl. Acad. Sci. USA 1997 Sep; 94:10367–10372
7. Pappa G, Strathmann J, Lowinger M, Bartsch H, Gerhauser C. Quantitative combination effects between sulforaphane and 3,3#-diindolylmethane on proliferation of human colon cancer cells in vitro. Carcinogenesis 2007, 28 (7):1471–1477
8. Vermeulen M, Ineke W. A. A. Klöpping-Ketelaars IWAA, Van den Berg R, Vaes WHJ. Bioavailability and Kinetics of Sulforaphane in Humans after Consumption of Cooked versus Raw Broccoli. J. Agric. Food Chem., 2008, 56 (22):10505–10509
9. Fowke JH, Chung F-L, Jin F, et al. Urinary Isothiocyanate Levels, Brassica, and Human Breast Cancer. Cancer Res 2003;63:3980-3986
10. Cornblatt BS, Ye L, Kostova AT, Erb M, Fahey JW, Singh NK,Chen M-SA, Stierer T, Garrett-Mayer E, Argani P, Davidson NE, Talalay P, Kensler TW, Visvanathan K. Preclinical and clinical evaluation of sulforaphane for chemoprevention in the breast. Carcinogenesis 2007;28 (7):1485–1490, 2007
11. Kensler TW, Chen J-G, Egner PA, et al. Effects of Glucosinolate-Rich Broccoli Sprouts on Urinary Levels of Aflatoxin-DNA Adducts and Phenanthrene Tetraols in a Randomized Clinical Trial in He Zuo Township, Qidong, People's Republic of China. Cancer Epidemiol Biomarkers Prev 2005;14:2605-2613.
12. Cohen JH, Kristal AR, Stanford JL. Fruit and Vegetable Intakes and Prostate Cancer Risk. Journal of the National Cancer Institute, 2000; 92 (1), Jan 5:61-68
13. Kolonel LN, Hankin JH, Whittemore AS, et al.Vegetables, Fruits, Legumes and Prostate Cancer: A Multiethnic Case-Control Study. Cancer Epidemiology, Biomarkers & Prevention 2000;9 (Aug):795–804
14. Broccoli sprouts in Wikipedia [ref to EH Jeffery unable to be found, but useful table]
15. Nechuta SJ, Shu OX of Vanderbilt-Ingram Cancer Center and Shanghai Center for Disease Control and Prevention. Results presented at the American Association for Cancer Research Annual Meeting in Chicago, Ill. Press release reported by Science Daily Apr. 3, 2012 (online)
16. Terry P, Wolk A, Persson I,Magnusson C. Brassica Vegetables and Breast Cancer Risk. JAMA, June 20, 2001;285(23):2975-2977
17. Bosetti C, Filomeno M, Riso P et al. Cruciferous vegetables and cancer risk in a network ofcase–control studies. Ann Oncol (2012) 23 (8): 2198-2203
18. Shapiro TA, Fahey JW, Wade KL, et al. Human metabolism and excretion of cancer chemoprotective glucosinolates and isothiocyanates of cruciferous vegetables. Cancer Epidemiol Biomarkers Prev 1998;7:1091–1100

19. Vermeulen M, Klöpping-Ketelaars IW, van den Berg R, Vaes WH. Bioavailability and kinetics of sulforaphane in humans after consumption of cooked versus raw broccoli. J Agric Food Chem. 2008 Nov 26;56(22):10505-9
20. Author's comments on her paper Ref #4 above. Quote retrieved from http://www.naturalnews.com/031498_broccoli_cancer.html
21. Erucic acid in food: A toxicological review and risk assessment. Technical report series No. 21. Published by Food Standards Australia New Zealand. June 30, available online
22. West L, Tsui I, Balch B, Meyer K, Huth PJ. Determination and Health Implication of the Erucic Acid Content of Broccoli Florets, Sprouts, and Seeds. Journal of Food Science 2006; 67(7):2641 – 2643
23. Minich DM, Position Paper on I3C and DIM. May 2004. http://www.metaproteomicslabs.com/
24. Zhang Y, Tang L. Discovery and development of sulforaphane as a cancer chemopreventive phytochemical. Acta Pharmacol Sin 2007;28 (9): 1343–1354
25. Gamet-Payrastre L. Signaling Pathways and Intracellular Targets of Sulforaphane Mediating Cell Cycle Arrest and Apoptosis. Current Cancer Drug Targets 2006; Mar; 6 (2):135-145
26. Khor TO, Keum YS, Lin W, Kim JH, Hu R, Shen G, Xu C, Gopalakrishnan A, Reddy B, Zheng X, Conney AH, Kong AN. Combined inhibitory effects of curcumin and phenethyl isothiocyanate on the growth of human PC-3 prostate xenografts in immunodeficient mice. Cancer Res. 2006 Jan 15;66(2):613-21
27. Ho E, Clarke JD, Dashwood RH. Dietary Sulforaphane, a Histone Deacetylase Inhibitor for Cancer Prevention. The Journal of Nutrition Dec 1, 2009:2393-2396
28. Le HT, Schaldach CM, Firestone GL, Bjeldanes LF. Plant-derived 3,3-Diindolylmethane Is a Strong Androgen Antagonist in Human Prostate Cancer Cells. J Biol Chem 2003 June; 278 (23):21136-21145
29. Muti P, Bradlow HL, Micheli A, Krogh V, Freudenheim JL et al. Estrogen Metabolism and Risk of Breast Cancer: A Prospective Study of the 2:16a-Hydroxyestrone Ratio in Premenopausal and Postmenopausal Women. Epidemiology 2000; 11(6):635-640
30. Fowke JH, Longcope C, Hebert JR. Brassica Vegetable Consumption Shifts Estrogen Metabolism in Healthy Postmenopausal Women Cancer Epidemiology, Biomarkers & Prevention Aug 2000; 9:773–779
31. Meng Q, Yuan F, Goldberg ID, Rosen EM, Auborn K, Fan S. Indole-3-Carbinol Is a Negative Regulator of Estrogen Receptor-a Signaling in Human Tumor Cells. J. Nutr. 2000;130(12):2927-2931
32. McGuire KP, Ngoubilly N, Neavyn M, Lanza-Jacoby S. 3,3'-diindolylmethane and paclitaxel act synergistically to promote apoptosis in HER2/Neu human breast cancer cells. J Surg Res. 2006 May 15;132(2):208-13
33. Wang XH, Cavell BE, Syed Alwi SS, Packham G. Inhibition of hypoxia inducible factor by phenethyl isothiocyanate. Biochem Pharmacol. 2009 Aug 1;78(3):261-72

34. Huang C, W-Y, LI J, Hecht SS, Dong Z. Essential Role of p53 in Phenethyl Isothiocyanate-induced Apoptosis. Cancer Res Sep 15, 1998; 58:4102
35. McGrath D, Frydoonfar H, Spigelman AD. Potential mechanisms for the chemopreventive effect of cruciferous vegetables in colorectal cancer: a clinical trial of indole-3-carbinol. Annals of Oncology (poster)2007 Supp 4 Vol 18; 410
36. Tang L, Zirpoli GR, Guru K, Moysich KB, Zhang Y, Ambrosone CB, McCann SE. Intake of cruciferous vegetables modifies bladder cancer survival. Cancer Epidemiol Biomarkers Prev. 2010 Jul;19(7):1806-11
37. Talalay P, Fahey JW, Healy ZR, Wehage SL et al. Sulforaphane mobilizes cellular defenses that protect skin against damage by UV radiation. Proc Natl Acad Sci U S A. 2007 Oct 30; 104(44): 17500–17505.

References for Chapters 2 and 21: Berries

1. God J, Tate PL, Larcom LL. Red raspberries have antioxidant effects that play a minor role in the killing of stomach and colon cancer cells. Nutr Res. 2010 Nov;30(11):777-82.
2. Stoner GD, Dombkowski AA, Reen RK, Cukovic D, Salagrama S, Wang L-S, Lechner JF. Carcinogen-Altered Genes in Rat Esophagus Positively Modulated to Normal Levels of Expression by Both Black Raspberries and Phenylethyl Isothiocyanate. Cancer Res 2008;68:6460-6467
3. Stoner GD. Foodstuffs for Preventing Cancer: The Preclinical and Clinical Development of Berries. Cancer Prev Res (Phila). 2009 Mar;2(3):187-194
4. Johnson SA, Arjmandi BH. Evidence for anti-cancer properties of blueberries: a mini-review. Anticancer Agents Med Chem 2013 Oct;13(8):1142-8
5. Seeram NP. Berry fruits for cancer prevention: current status and future prospects. J Agric Food Chem. 2008 Feb 13;56(3):630-5
6. BI X, Fang W, Wang LS, Stoner GD, Yang W. Black raspberries inhibit intestinal tumorigenesis in apc1638+/- and Muc2-/- mouse models of colorectal cancer. Cancer Prev Res (Phila). 2010 Nov;3(11):1443-50
7. Casto BC, Kresty LA, Kraly CL, Pearl DK, Knobloch TJ, Schut HA, Stoner GD, Mallery SR, Weghorst CM. Chemoprevention of oral cancer by black raspberries. Anticancer Res. 2002 Nov-Dec;22(6C):4005-15
8. Wang LS, Hecht SS, Carmella SG, Yu N, Larue B, Henry C, McIntyre C, Rocha C, Lechner JF, Stoner GD. Anthocyanins in black raspberries prevent esophageal tumors in rats. Cancer Prev Res (Phila). 2009 Jan;2(1):84-93
9. Olsson ME, Andersson CS, Oredsson S, Berglund RH, Gustavsson KE. Antioxidant levels and inhibition of cancer cell proliferation in vitro by extracts from organically and conventionally cultivated strawberries. J Agric Food Chem. 2006 Feb 22;54(4):1248-55.
10. Nixon D. Alternative and Complementary Therapies in Oncology Care. J Clin Onc 1999Nov Vol 17 Suppl 1:35-37
11. Liu M, LI XQ, Weber C, Lee CY, Brown J, Liu RH. Antioxidant and antiproliferative activities of raspberries. J Agric Food Chem 2002 May 8;50(10):2926-30

12. Olsson ME, Gustavsson KE, Andersson S, Nilsson A, Duan RD. Inhibition of cancer cell proliferation in vitro by fruit and berry extracts and correlations with antioxidant levels. J Agric Food Chem. 2004 Dec 1;52(24):7264-71
13. Chen T, Yan F, Qian J, Guo M, Zhang H, Tang X, Chen F, Stoner GD, Wang X. Randomized phase II trial of lyophilized strawberries in patients with dysplastic precancerous lesions of the esophagus. Cancer Prev Res (Phila). 2012 Jan;5(1):41-50
14. Colditz GA, Branch LG, Lipnick RJ et al. Increased green and yellow vegetable intake and lowered cancer deaths in an elderly population. Am J Clin Nutr 1985 Jan 41:32-36
15. Liu M, LI XQ, Weber C, Lee CY, Brown J, Liu RH. Antioxidant and antiproliferative activities of raspberries. J Agric Food Chem. 2002 May 8;50(10):2926-30
16. Daniel EM, Krupnick AD, Heur Y-H, Blinzler JS, Nims RE, Stoner GD. Extraction, stability, and quantitation of ellagic acid in various fruits and nuts. J.Food Comp and Anal 1989;2:338–49
17. Shailendra K. Pterostilbene and its emerging antineoplastic effects: a prospective treatment option for systemic malignancies. Am J Surg 2013Apr 205.4 :483
18. McCormack D, Schneider J, McDonald D, McFadden D. The antiproliferative effects of pterostilbene on breast cancer in vitro are via inhibition of constitutive and leptin-induced Janus kinase/signal transducer and activator of transcription activation. Am J Surg 2011 202:541–544
19. Barak V, Halperin T, Kalickman I. The effect of Sambucol, a black elderberry-based, natural product, on the production of human cytokines: I. Inflammatory cytokines. Eur Cyto Network 2001Jun;12(2):290-6
20. Elderberry. Retrieved from http://www.mskcc.org/cancer-care/herb/elderberry-0
21. Thole JM, Kraft TF, Sueiro LA, Kang YH, Gills JJ, Cuendet M, Pezzuto JM, Seigler DS, Lila MA. A comparative evaluation of the anticancer properties of European and American elderberry fruits. J Med Food 2006 Winter;9(4):498-504
22. González-Barrio R, Borges G, Mullen W, Crozier A. Bioavailability of anthocyanins and ellagitannins following consumption of raspberries by healthy humans and subjects with an ileostomy. J Agric Food Chem. 2010 Apr 14;58(7):3933-9
23. Heber D. Multitargeted therapy of cancer by ellagitannins. Cancer Lett. 2008 Oct 8;269(2):262-8
24. Black raspberries show multiple defenses in thwarting cancer. Retrieved from http://researchnews.osu.edu/archive/canberry.htm (Dr Gary Stoner quoted, Ref#3 above)
25. Debunking 3 black raspberry myths. Retrieved from http://www.blackraspberrybuzz.com/debunking-3-black-raspberry-capsule-myths
26. Mertens-Talcott SU, Percival SS. Ellagic acid and quercetin interact synergistically with resveratrol in the induction of apoptosis and cause

transient cell cycle arrest in human leukemia cells. Cancer Lett. 2005 Feb 10;218(2):141-51

27. Mertens-Talcott SU, Talcott ST, Percival SS. Low concentrations of quercetin and ellagic acid synergistically influence proliferation, cytotoxicity and apoptosis in MOLT-4 human leukemia cells. J Nutr 2003 Aug;133(8):2669-74

References for Chapters 3 and 22: Turmeric

(also see Chapter 18 refs 17-21)

1. Cancer rates India versus USA. Retrieved from http://www.mightyturmeric.com/80/cancer-rates-india-versus-us/
2. Garcea G, Jones DJ, Singh R, Dennison AR et al. Detection of curcumin and its metabolites in hepatic tissue and portal blood of patients following oral administration. Br J Cancer 2004; 90(5):1011–5
3. Cruz-Correa M, Shoskes DA, Sanchez P, Zhao R et al. Combination treatment with curcumin and quercetin of adenomas in familial adenomatous polyposis. Clin Gastroenterol Hepatol 2006;4(8):1035–8
4. Turmeric adds spice to your health. Retrieved from http://www2.mdanderson.org/cancerwise/2011/01/turmeric-adds-spice-to-your-health.html
5. Du Q, Hu B, An HM, Shen KP, Xu L, Deng S, Wei MM. Synergistic anticancer effects of curcumin and resveratrol in Hepa1-6 hepatocellular carcinoma cells. Oncol Rep. 2013 May;29(5):1851-8
6. Khafif A, Schantz SP, Chou TC, Edelstein D, Sacks PG. Quantitation of chemopreventive synergism between (-)-epigallocatechin-3-gallate and curcumin in normal, premalignant and malignant human oral epithelial cells. Carcinogenesis. 1998 Mar;19(3):419-24
7. Parasramka MA, Gupta SV. Synergistic effect of garcinol and curcumin on antiproliferative and apoptotic activity in pancreatic cancer cells. J Oncol 2012;2012:709739
8. Cheng AL, Hsu CH, Lin JK, Hsu MM, et al. Phase I clinical trial of curcumin, a chemopreventive agent, in patients with high-risk or pre-malignant lesions. Anticancer Res 2001 Jul-Aug;21(4B):2895-900
9. Singh S, Khar A. Biological effects of curcumin and its role in cancer chemoprevention and therapy. Anticancer Agents Med Chem. 2006 May;6(3):259-70
10. Lee CK, KI SH, Choi JS. Effects of oral curcumin on the pharmacokinetics of intravenous and oral etoposide in rats: possible role of intestinal CYP3A and P-gp inhibition by curcumin. Biopharm Drug Dispos 2011 May;32(4):245-51
11. Duarte VM, Han E, Veena MS, Salvado A, Suh JD, Liang LJ, Faull KF, Srivatsan ES, Wang MB. Curcumin enhances the effect of cisplatin in suppression of head and neck squamous cell carcinoma via inhibition of IKKβ protein of the NFκB pathway. Mol Cancer Ther 2010 Oct;9(10):2665-75
12. Bava SV, Puliappadamba VT, Deepti A, Nair A, Karunagaran D, Anto RJ. Sensitization of taxol-induced apoptosis by curcumin involves

down-regulation of nuclear factor-kappaB and the serine/threonine kinase Akt and is independent of tubulin polymerization. J Biol Chem 2005 Feb 25;280(8):6301-8

13. Somasundaram S, Edmund NA, Moore DT, Small GW, Shi YY, Orlowski RZ. Dietary curcumin inhibits chemotherapy-induced apoptosis in models of human breast cancer. Cancer Res 2002 Jul 1;62(13):3868-75
14. Anand P, Kunnumakkara AB, Newman RA, Aggarwal BB. Bioavailability of Curcumin: Problems and Promises. Mol Pharmaceutics, 2007;4(6):807-818
15. Shoba G, Joy D, Joseph T, Majeed M, Rajendran R, Srinivas PS. Influence of piperine on the pharmacokinetics of curcumin in animals and human volunteers. Planta Med 1998 May;64(4):353-6
16. Srinivasan K. Black pepper and its pungent principle-piperine: a review of diverse physiological effects. Crit Rev Food Sci Nutr 2007;47(8):735-48
17. Kakarala M, Brenner DE, Khorkaya H, Cheng C et al. Targeting Breast Stem Cells with the Cancer Preventive Compounds Curcumin and Piperine. Breast Cancer Res Treat 2010 Aug; 122(3):777–785

References for Chapters 4 and 23: Garlic

1. Weiner L, Shin I, Shimon LJ, Miron T, Wilchek M, Mirelman D, Frolow F, Rabinkov A. Thiol-disulfide organization in alliin lyase (alliinase) from garlic (Allium sativum). Protein Sci 2009 Jan;18(1):196-205
2. Lawson LD. in Human Medicinal Agents from Plants. 1993;Ch 21(Bioactive organosulfur compounds of garlic and garlic products):306–330
3. Song K, Milner JA. The influence of heating on the anticancer properties of garlic. J Nutr 2001 Mar;131(3s):1054S-7S
4. Lawson LD, Hughes BG. Characterization of the formation of allicin and other thiosulfinates from garlic. Planta Med. 1992 Aug;58(4):345-50
5. Slimestad R, Fossen T, Vagen IM. Onions: A Source of Unique Dietary Flavonoids. J Agric Food Chem 2007;55 (25):10067-10080
6. Yang J, Meyers KJ, van der Heide J, Liu RH. Varietal Differences in Phenolic Content and Antioxidant and Antiproliferative Activities of Onions. J Agric Food Chem 2004;52(22):6787-6793
7. Song JD, Lee SK, Kim KM, Park SE, Park SJ, Kim KH, Ahn SC, Park YC. Molecular mechanism of diallyl disulfide in cell cycle arrest and apoptosis in HCT-116 colon cancer cells. J Biochem Mol Toxicol 2009 Jan-Feb;23(1):71-9
8. Mendoza EE, Burd R. Quercetin as a systemic chemopreventative agent: structural and functional mechanisms. Mini Rev Med Chem 2011 Dec;11(14):1216-21
9. Wang L-S, Stoner GD. Anthocyanins and their role in cancer prevention. Cancer Lett. 2008 Oct 8; 269(2):281–290
10. Sivam GP. Protection against Helicobacter pylori and other bacterial infections by garlic. J Nutr 2001 Mar;131(3s):1106S-8S
11. Gorinstein S, Leontowicz H, Leontowicz M, Namiesnik J. Comparison of the Main Bioactive Compounds and Antioxidant Activities in Garlic and

White and Red Onions after Treatment Protocols. J Agric Food Chem 2008;56(12):4418-4426

12. Xiao D, Pinto JT, Soh JW, Deguchi A, Gundersen GG, Palazzo AF, Yoon JT, Shirin H, Weinstein IB. Induction of apoptosis by the garlic-derived compound S-allylmercaptocysteine (SAMC) is associated with microtubule depolymerization and c-Jun NH(2)-terminal kinase 1 activation. Cancer Res 2003 Oct 15;63(20):6825-37
13. Galeone C, Pelucchi C, Levi F, Negri E, Franceschi S, Talamini R, Giacosa A, La Vecchia C. Onion and garlic use and human cancer. Am J Clin Nutr 2006 Nov;84(5):1027-32
14. Steinmetz KA, Kushi LH, Bostick RM, Folsom AR, Potter JD. Vegetables, fruit, and colon cancer in the Iowa Women's Health Study. Am J Epidemiol 1994 Jan 1;139(1):1-15
15. Piscitelli SC, Burstein AH, Welden N, Gallicano KD, Falloon J. The effect of garlic supplements on the pharmacokinetics of saquinavir. Clinical Infectious Diseases 2002;34(2):234-238
16. Kim JY, Kwon O. Garlic intake and cancer risk: an analysis using the Food and Drug Administration's evidence-based review system for the scientific evaluation of health claims. Am J Clin Nutr 2009 Jan;89(1):257-64
17. Tsubura A, Lai YC, Kuwata M, Uehara N, Yoshizawa K. Anticancer effects of garlic and garlic-derived compounds for breast cancer control. Anticancer Agents Med Chem 2011 Mar;11(3):249-53
18. Hernandez LG, Forkert PG. Inhibition of vinyl carbamate-induced lung tumors and Kras2 mutations by the garlic derivative diallyl sulfone. Mutation Research/Fundamental and Molecular Mechanisms of Mutagenesis 2009 Mar;662,(1-2):16-21
19. Liu CT, Su HM, Lii CK, Sheen LY. Effect of supplementation with garlic oil on activity of Th1 and Th2 lymphocytes from rats. Planta Med 2009 Feb;75(3):205-10
20. Lamson DW, Brignall MS. Antioxidants and Cancer III: Quercetin. Alternative Medicine Review 2000;5(3):196-208
21. Fleischauer AT, Arab L. Garlic and cancer: a critical review of the epidemiologic literature. J Nutr 2001 Mar;131(3s):1032S-40S
22. You W, Blot WJ, Chang Y, Ershow AG et al. Allium vegetables and reduced risk of stomach cancer. J Natl Cancer Inst 1989;81:162-164
23. Le Marchand L, Hankin JH, Wilkens LR, Kolonel LN, Englyst HN, Lyu LC. Dietary fiber and colorectal cancer risk. Epidemiology 1997;8:658–665
24. McCullough ML, Jacobs EJ, Shah R, Campbell PT, Gapstur SM.Abstract B101: Garlic consumption and colorectal cancer risk in the CPS-II Nutrition Cohort. Cancer Prev Res 2011;4(10 Suppl):B101
25. Fleischauer AT, Poole C, Arab L. Garlic consumption and cancer prevention: meta-analyses of colorectal and stomach cancers. Am J Clin Nutr 2000 Oct;72(4):1047-52
26. Chan JM, Wang F, Holly EA. Vegetable and fruit intake and pancreatic cancer in a population-based case-control study in the San Francisco bay area. Cancer Epidemiology Biomarkers & Prevention 2005;14(9):2093-2097

27. Challier B, Perarnau JM, Viel JF. Garlic, onion and cereal fibre as protective factors for breast cancer: A French case-control study. European Journal of Epidemiology 1998;14(8):737-747
28. National Cancer Institute Factsheet http://www.cancer.gov/cancertopics/factsheet/prevention/garlic-and-cancer-prevention

References for Chapters 5 and 24: Green tea (and coffee)

1. Boehm K, Borrelli F, Ernst E, Habacher G, Hung SK, Milazzo S, Horneber M. Green tea (Camellia sinensis) for the prevention of cancer (Review). In The Cochrane Collaboration. 2010, Issue 1. Published by JohnWiley & Sons, Ltd.
2. Lorenz M, Jochmann N, von Krosigk A, Martus P, Baumann G, Stangl K, Stangl V. Addition of milk prevents vascular protective effects of tea European Heart Journal 2007;28:219-223
3. Green tea catechins. Retrieved from http://examine.com/supplements/Green+Tea+Catechins/#summary4
4. Decaffeination, green tea and benefits. Retrieved from http://www.teasetc.com/tea/article.asp?ID=3
5. Arts I, Van De Putte B, Hollman O. Catechins contents of foods commonly consumed, in the Netherlands. Tea, wine, fruit juices, and chocolate milk. J Agric Food Chem 2000;48:1752- 1757
6. Wang LF, Kim DM, Park JD, Lee CY. Various antibrowning agents and green tea extract during processing and storage. J Food Process Pres 2003;27:213-225
7. Bhagwat S, Haytowitz DB, Holden JM. USDA Database for the Flavonoid Content of Selected Foods. U.S. Department of Agriculture. Release 3.1, Dec 2013 (available online)
8. Khokhar S, Magnusdottir SG. Total phenol, catechin, and caffeine contents of teas commonly consumed in the United kingdom. J Agric Food Chem 2002 Jan 30;50(3):565-70
9. Shishikura Y, Khokhar S.Factors affecting the levels of catechins and caffeine in tea beverage: estimated daily intakes and antioxidant activity. J Sci Food Agric 2000;85:2125-2133
10. Peters CM, Green RJ, Janle EM, Ferruzzi MG. Formulation with ascorbic acid and sucrose modulates catechin bioavailability from green tea. Food Res Int 2010 January 1;43(1):95-102
11. Chow HS, Hakim IA, Vining DR et al. Effects of Dosing Condition on the Oral Bioavailability of Green Tea Catechins after Single-Dose Administration of Polyphenon E in Healthy Individuals. Clin Cancer Res 2005;11:4627-4633
12. Green RJ, Murphy AS, Schulz B, Watkins BA, Ferruzzi MG. Common tea formulations modulate in vitro digestive recovery of green tea catechins. Mol Nutr Food Res 2007 Sep;51(9):1152-62
13. Manikandan R, Beulaja M, Arulvasu C, Sellamuthu S, Dinesh D, Prabhu D, Babu G, Vaseeharan B, Prabhu NM. Synergistic anticancer activity of

curcumin and catechin: an in vitro study using human cancer cell lines. Microsc Res Tech 2012 Feb;75(2):112-6

14. Su YL, Leung LK, Huang Y, Chen Z-Y. Stability of tea theaflavins and catechins. Food Chemistry 2003 Nov;83(2):189–195
15. Chen Z-Y, Zhu QY, Wong YF, Zhang Z, Chung HY. Stabilizing Effect of Ascorbic Acid on Green Tea Catechins. J Agric Food Chem 1998;46(7):2512-2516
16. Huang M-T, Xie J-G, Wang ZY et al. Effects of Tea, Decaffeinated Tea, and Caffeine on UVB Light-induced Complete Carcinogenesis in SKH-1 Mice: Demonstration of Caffeine as a Biologically Important Constitutent of Tea. Cancer Research 1997 July 1;57:2623-2629
17. Tuntawiroon M. Dose-dependent inhibitory effect of phenolic compounds in foods on non-heme iron absorption in men. Am J Clin Nutr 1991;53:554-557
18. Flaten TP. Aluminum in tea concentrations, speciation and bioavailability. Coordin Chem Rev 2002;228:385-395
19. Higdon JV, Frei B. Tea catechins and polyphenols: health effects, metabolism, and antioxidant functions. Crit Rev Food Sci Nutr 2003;43:89-143
20. Sala M, Cordier S, Chang-Claude J, et al. Coffee consumption and bladder cancer in nonsmokers: a pooled analysis of case-control studies in European countries. Cancer Causes Control 2000;11(10):925-31
21. Pelucchi C, Tavani A, Negri E, Franceschi S, La Vecchia C. Tobacco smoking and bladder cancer in coffee non-drinkers. J Epidemiol Community Health 2002;56:78-79
22. LI XJ, Ren ZJ, Qin JW, Zhao JH, Tang JH, JI MH, Wu JZ. Coffee consumption and risk of breast cancer: an up-to-date meta-analysis. PLoS One 2013;8(1):e52681
23. Simonsson M, Söderlind V, Henningson M, Hjertberg M, Rose C, Ingvar C, Jernström H. Coffee prevents early events in tamoxifen-treated breast cancer patients and modulates hormone receptor status. Cancer Causes Control 2013 May;24(5):929-40
24. Je Y, Hankinson SE, Tworoger SS, De Vivo I, Giovannucci E. A prospective cohort study of coffee consumption and risk of endometrial cancer over a 26-year follow-up. Cancer Epidemiol Biomarkers Prev 2011 Dec;20(12):2487-95
25. Wilson KM, Kasperzyk JL, Rider JR, Kenfield S, van Dam RM, Stampfer MJ, Giovannucci E, Mucci LA. Coffee consumption and prostate cancer risk and progression in the Health Professionals Follow-up Study. J Natl Cancer Inst 2011 Jun 8;103(11):876-84
26. Yu X, Bao Z, Zou J, Dong J. Coffee consumption and risk of cancers: a meta-analysis of cohort studies. BMC Cancer 2011;11: 96
27. Nakachi K, Suemasu K, Suga K, Takeo T, Imai K, Higashi Y. Influence of drinking green tea on breast cancer malignancy among Japanese patients. Jpn J Cancer Res 1998 Mar;89(3):254-61

28. Kumar N, Titus-Ernstoff L, Newcomb P, Trentham-Dietz, Anic G, Egan KM. Tea Consumption and Risk of Breast Cancer. Cancer Epidemiol Biomarkers Prev Jan 2009;18:341
29. Bettuzzi S, Brausi M, Rizzi F et al. Chemoprevention of Human Prostate Cancer by Oral Administration of Green Tea Catechins in Volunteers with High-Grade Prostate Intraepithelial Neoplasia: A Preliminary Report from a One-Year Proof-of-Principle Study. Cancer Res January 15, 2006;66:1234
30. Wu AH, Yu MC, Tseng CC, Hankin J, Pike MC. Green tea and risk of breast cancer in Asian Americans. Int J Cancer 2003 Sep 10;106(4):574-9
31. Ogunleye AA, Xue F, Michels KB. Green tea consumption and breast cancer risk or recurrence: a meta-analysis. Breast Cancer Res Treat 2010 Jan;119(2):477-84
32. Inoue M, Tajima K, Mizutani M, Iwata H, Iwase T, Miura S, Hirose K, Hamajima N, Tominaga S. Regular consumption of green tea and the risk of breast cancer recurrence: follow-up study from the Hospital-based Epidemiologic Research Program at Aichi Cancer Center (HERPACC), Japan. Cancer Lett 2001 Jun 26;167(2):175-82
33. Sun C-L, Yuan J-M, Lee M-J, Yang CS et al.Urinary tea polyphenols in relation to gastric and esophageal cancers: a prospective study of men in Shanghai, China. Carcinogenesis 2002;23(9):1497-1503
34. Nechuta S, Shu X-O, LI H-L, Yang G et al. Prospective cohort study of tea consumption and risk of digestive system cancers: results from the Shanghai Women's Health Study. Am J Clin Nutr Nov 2012;96(5):1056-1063
35. LI N, Sun Z, Han C, Chen J. The chemopreventive effects of tea on human oral precancerous mucosa lesions. Proceedings from the Society of Experimental Biology and Medicine 1999; 220(4):218–224
36. Luo H, Tang L, Tang M, et al. Phase IIa chemoprevention trial of green tea polyphenols in high-risk individuals of liver cancer: Modulation of urinary excretion of green tea polyphenols and 8-hydroxydeoxyguanosine. Carcinogenesis 2006; 27(2):262-268
37. Jia Y, Hu T, Hang CY, Yang R, LI X, Chen ZL, Mei YD, Zhang QH, Huang KC, Xiang QY et al. Case-control study of diet in patients with cervical cancer or precancerosis in Wufeng, a high incidence region in China. Asian Pac J Cancer Prev 2012;13(10):5299-302
38. Wang X, Lin YW, Wang S, Wu J, Mao QQ, Zheng XY, Xie LP. A meta-analysis of tea consumption and the risk of bladder cancer. Urol Int 2013;90(1):10-6
39. Wang XJ, Zeng XT, Duan XL, Zeng HC, Shen R, Zhou P. Association between green tea and colorectal cancer risk: a meta-analysis of 13 case-control studies. Asian Pac J Cancer Prev 2012;13(7):3123-7
40. Davalli P, Rizzi F, Caporali A, Pellacani D et al. Anticancer Activity of Green Tea Polyphenols in Prostate Gland. Oxid Med Cell Longev 2012;2012:984219
41. Kanwar J, Taskeen M, Mohammad I, Huo C et al. Recent advances on tea polyphenols. Front Biosci (Elite Ed). 2012 Jan 1;4:111-131

42. Beltz LA, Bayer DK, Moss AL, Simet IM. Mechanisms of cancer prevention by green and black tea polyphenols. Anticancer Agents Med Chem 2006 Sep;6(5):389-406
43. Cabrera C, Artacho R, Giménez R. Beneficial effects of green tea--a review. J Am Coll Nutr 2006 Apr;25(2):79-99
44. Rodriguez SK, Guo W, Liu L, Band MA, Paulson EK, Meydani M. Green tea catechin, epigallocatechin-3-gallate, inhibits vascular endothelial growth factor angiogenic signaling by disrupting the formation of a receptor complex. Int J Cancer 2006 Apr 1;118(7):1635-44
45. Jung Y, Ellis LM. Inhibition of tumour invasion and angiogenesis by epigallocatechin gallate (EGCG), a major component of green tea. Int J Exp Pathol 2001 Dec; 82(6):309-316
46. Liu L, Lai C-Q, Nie L, Ordovas J et al. The Modulation of Endothelial Cell Gene Expression By Green Tea Polyphenol-EGCG. Mol Nutr Food Res 2008 Oct; 52(10):1182-1192
47. Devine A, Hodgson JM, Dick IM, Prince RL. Tea drinking is associated with benefits on bone density in older women. Am J Clin Nutr 2007;86:1243-7
48. Hegarty VM, May HM, Khaw K-T. Tea drinking and bone mineral density in older women. Am J Clin Nutr 2000;71:1003-7

References for Chapters 6 and 25: Flaxseeds

1. Candela CG, López LMB, Kohen VL. Importance of a balanced omega 6/omega 3 ratio for the maintenance of health. Nutritional recommendations. Nutr Hosp. 2011;26(2):323-329
2. Rose DP. Dietary fatty acids and cancer. Am J Clin Nutr 1997;66(suppl): 998S-1003S
3. Milder IEJ, Arts ICW, van de Putte B, Venema DP, Hollman PCH. Lignan contents of Dutch plant foods: a database including lariciresinol, pinoresinol, secoisolariciresinol and matairesinol. British Journal of Nutrition 2005;93:393-402
4. Pregnant women consuming flaxseed have a high risk of premature birth. Retrieved from http://www.eurekalert.org/pub_releases/2008-10/uom-pwc102708.php (unpublished study from Université de Montréal (Berard A, Moussally K)
5. Vinikoor LC, Schroeder JC, Millikan RC, Satia JA, Martin CF, Ibrahim J, Galanko JA, Sandler RS. Consumption of trans-fatty acid and its association with colorectal adenomas. Am J Epidemiol 2008 Aug 1;168(3):289-97
6. Slattery ML, Benson J, Ma KN, Schaffer D, Potter JD. Trans-fatty acids and colon cancer. Nutr Cancer 2001;39(2):170-5
7. Thompson AK, Shaw DI, Minihane AM, Williams CM. Trans-fatty acids and cancer: the evidence reviewed. Nutrition Research Reviews 2008;21:174-188
8. Lipworth L, Sonderman JS, Tarone RE, McLaughlin JK. Review of epidemiologic studies of dietary acrylamide intake and the risk of cancer. Eur J Cancer Prev 2012 Jul;21(4):375-86

9. Omega 3 fatty acids. Retrieved from http://www.whfoods.com/genpage.php?tname=nutrient&dbid=84#foodchart
10. Ponnampalam EN, Mann NJ, Sinclair AJ. Effect of feeding systems on omega-3 fatty acids, conjugated linoleic acid and trans fatty acids in Australian beef cuts: potential impact on human health. Asia Pac J Clin Nutr 2006;15(1):21-9
11. Lee KW, Lee HJ, Cho HY, Kim YJ. Role of the conjugated linoleic acid in the prevention of cancer. Crit Rev Food Sci Nutr 2005;45(2):135-44
12. Horrobin DF. Fatty acid metabolism in health and disease: the role of delta-6-desaturase. Am J Clin Nutr 1993; 57(suppl):732S-737S
13. Understanding eicosanoids. Retrieved from http://www.drsears.com/ArticlePreview/tabid/399/itemid/66/Default.aspx
14. Horrobin DF. Loss of delta-6-desaturase activity as a key factor in aging. Med Hypotheses 1981 Sep;7(9):1211-20
15. Brasky TM, Lampe JW, Potter JD, et al. Specialty Supplements and Breast Cancer Risk in the VITamins And Lifestyle (VITAL) Cohort. Cancer Epidemiol Biomarkers Prev 2010;19:1696-1708
16. Simopoulos AP. Essential fatty acids in health and chronic disease. Am J Clin Nutr 1999;70(suppl):560S-9S
17. Comparing Omega 3s from fish and flax seed oil. Retrieved from http://www.omega3sealoil.com/Chapter4_3c.html
18. Stoll BA. N-3 fatty acids and lipid peroxidation in breast cancer inhibition. Br J Nutr 2002 Mar;87(3):193-8
19. Bhatia E, Doddivenaka C, Zhang X, Bommareddy A, Krishnan P, Matthees DP, Dwivedi C. Chemopreventive effects of dietary canola oil on colon cancer development. Nutr Cancer 2011 Feb;63(2):242-7
20. Bommareddy A, Arasada BL, Mathees DP, Dwivedi C. Chemopreventive effects of dietary flaxseed on colon tumor development. Nutr Cancer 2006;54(2):216-22
21. Mandal CC, Ghosh-Choudhury T, Yoneda T, Choudhury GG, Ghosh-Choudhury N. Fish oil prevents breast cancer cell metastasis to bone. Biochem Biophys Res Commun 2010 Nov 26;402(4):602-7
22. Hardman WE. Walnuts Have Potential for Cancer Prevention and Treatment in Mice. J Nutr 2014 Feb 5. [Epub ahead of print]
23. Perinatal Nutrition Working Group, a program of the National Healthy Mothers, Healthy Babies Coalition (White paper). Benefits of Seafood Consumption and Omega-3 DHA During Pregnancy and Early Post-Natal Development. March 2012 (available online)
24. Touvier M, Kesse-Guyot E, Andreeva VA, Fezeu L et al. Modulation of the association between plasma intercellular adhesion molecule-1 and cancer risk by n23 PUFA intake: a nested case-control study. Am J Clin Nutr 2012 Apr;95(4):944-50
25. Maillard V, Bougnoux P, Ferrari P, Jourdan ML, Pinault M, Lavillonnière F, Body G, Le Floch O, Chajès V. N-3 and N-6 fatty acids in breast adipose tissue and relative risk of breast cancer in a case-control study in Tours, France. Int J Cancer 2002 Mar 1;98(1):78-83

26. Williams CD, Whitley BM, Hoyo C, Grant DJ, Iraggi JD, Newman KA, Gerber L, Taylor LA, McKeever MG, Freedland SJ. A high ratio of dietary n-6/n-3 polyunsaturated fatty acids is associated with increased risk of prostate cancer. Nutr Res 2011 Jan;31(1):1-8
27. Brasky TM, Till C, White E, Neuhouser ML, Song X, Goodman P, Thompson IM, King IB, Albanes D, Kristal AR. Serum phospholipid fatty acids and prostate cancer risk: results from the prostate cancer prevention trial. Am J Epidemiol 2011 Jun 15;173(12):1429-39
28. Euler L. Cancer Defeated Newsletter 257. Retrieved from http://www.cancerdefeated.com/omega-3-oils-good-for-breasts-bad-for-prostates/1385/
29. Pauwels EK. The protective effect of the Mediterranean diet: focus on cancer and cardiovascular risk. Med Princ Pract 2011;20(2):103-11
30. Simopoulos AP. The traditional diet of Greece and cancer. Eur J Cancer Prev 2004 Jun;13(3):219-30
31. Cui PH, Petrovic N, Murray M. The ω-3 epoxide of eicosapentaenoic acid inhibits endothelial cell proliferation by p38 MAP kinase activation and cyclin D1/CDK4 down-regulation. Br J Pharmacol 2011 Mar;162(5):1143-55
32. Mita R, Beaulieu MJ, Field C, Godbout R. Brain fatty acid-binding protein and omega-3/omega-6 fatty acids: mechanistic insight into malignant glioma cell migration. J Biol Chem 2010 Nov 19;285(47):37005-15
33. Keijer J, Bekkenkamp-Grovenstein M, Venema D, Dommels YE. Bioactive food components, cancer cell growth limitation and reversal of glycolytic metabolism. Biochim Biophys Acta 2011 Jun;1807(6):697-706
34. Kang JX, Liu A. The role of the tissue omega-6/omega-3 fatty acid ratio in regulating tumor angiogenesis. Cancer Metastasis Rev. 2013 Jun;32(1-2):201-10
35. Menendez JA, Vazquez-Martin A, Garcia-Villalba R, Carrasco-Pancorbo A, Oliveras-Ferraros C, Fernandez-Gutierrez A, Segura-Carretero A. tabAnti-HER2 (erbB-2) oncogene effects of phenolic compounds directly isolated from commercial Extra-Virgin Olive Oil (EVOO). BMC Cancer 2008 Dec 18;8:377
36. Chang CS, Sun HL, Lii CK, Chen HW, Chen PY, Liu KL. Gamma-linolenic acid inhibits inflammatory responses by regulating NF-kappaB and AP-1 activation in lipopolysaccharide-induced RAW 264.7 macrophages. Inflammation 2010 Feb;33(1):46-57
37. Thompson LU, Chen JM, LI T, Strasser-Weippl K, Goss PE. Dietary flaxseed alters tumor biological markers in postmenopausal breast cancer. Clin Cancer Res 2005 May 15;11(10):3828-35
38. Buck K, Vrieling A, Zaineddin AK, Becker S, Hüsing A, Kaaks R, Linseisen J, Flesch-Janys D, Chang-Claude J. Serum enterolactone and prognosis of postmenopausal breast cancer. J Clin Oncol 2011 Oct 1;29(28):3730-8
39. Patterson RE. Flaxseed and breast cancer: what should we tell our patients? J Clin Oncol 2011 Oct 1;29(28):3723-4
40. Cotterchio M, Boucher BA, Manno M, Gallinger S, Okey A, Harper P. Dietary Phytoestrogen Intake Is Associated with Reduced Colorectal Cancer Risk. J Nutr 2006 Dec; 136:3046-3053

41. Kuijsten A, Arts IC, Hollman PC, van't Veer P, Kampman E. Plasma enterolignans are associated with lower colorectal adenoma risk. Cancer Epidemiol Biomarkers Prev 2006 Jun;15(6):1132-6
42. Hedelin M, Klint A, Chang ET, et al. Dietary phytoestrogen, serum enterolactone and risk of prostate cancer: the cancer prostate Sweden study (Sweden). Cancer Causes Control 2006 Mar;17(2):169-80
43. Heald CL, Ritchie MR, Bolton-Smith C, Morton MS, Alexander FE. Phyto-oestrogens and risk of prostate cancer in Scottish men. Br J Nutr 2007 Aug;98(2):388-96
44. McCann SE, Ambrosone CB, Moysich KB, et al. Intakes of selected nutrients, foods, and phytochemicals and prostate cancer risk in western New York. Nutr Cancer 2005;53(1):33-41
45. Chen J, Stavro PM, Thompson LU. Dietary flaxseed inhibits human breast cancer growth and metastasis and downregulates expression of insulin-like growth factor and epidermal growth factor receptor. Nutr Cancer 2002;43(2):187-92
46. Dabrosin C, Chen J, Wang L, Thompson LU. Flaxseed inhibits metastasis and decreases extracellular vascular endothelial growth factor in human breast cancer xenografts. Cancer Lett 2002 Nov 8;185(1):31-7
47. Evans BA, Griffiths K, Morton MS. Inhibition of 5 alpha-reductase in genital skin fibroblasts and prostate tissue by dietary lignans and isoflavonoids. J Endocrinol 1995 Nov;147(2):295-302
48. Denis L, Morton MS, Griffiths K. Diet and its preventive role in prostatic disease. Eur Urol 1999;35(5-6):377-87
49. Bergman JM, Thompson LU, Dabrosin C. Flaxseed and its lignans inhibit estradiol-induced growth, angiogenesis, and secretion of vascular endothelial growth factor in human breast cancer xenografts in vivo. Clin Cancer Res 2007 Feb 1;13(3):1061-7

References for Chapters 7 and 26: Mushrooms

1. Patel S, Goyal A. Recent developments in mushrooms as anti-cancer therapeutics: a review. 3 Biotech 2012 Mar;2(1):1-15
2. Medicinal mushrooms research – history, principles and results. Retrieved from http://www.mykosan.com/medicinal-mushroom-research.html (Myko San Medicinal Mushroom Research)
3. Ganeshpurkar A, Rai G, Jain AP. Medicinal mushrooms: Towards a new horizon. Pharmacogn Rev 2010 Jul-Dec;4(8):127-135
4. Hong SA, Kim K, Nam SJ, Kong G, Kim MK. A case-control study on the dietary intake of mushrooms and breast cancer risk among Korean women. Int J Cancer 2008 Feb 15;122(4):919-23
5. Liu X, Yuan JP, Chung CK, Chen XJ. Antitumor activity of the sporoderm-broken germinating spores of Ganoderma lucidum. Cancer Lett 2002 Aug 28;182(2):155-61
6. Sliva D, Labarrere C, Slivova V, Sedlak M, Lloyd FP Jr, Ho NW. Ganoderma lucidum suppresses motility of highly invasive breast and prostate cancer cells. Biochem Biophys Res Commun 2002 Nov 8;298(4):603-12

7. Konno S. Synergistic potentiation of D-fraction with vitamin C as possible alternative approach for cancer therapy. Int J Gen Med 2009 Jul 30;2:91-108
8. Brown DC, Reetz J. Single agent polysaccharopeptide delays metastases and improves survival in naturally occurring hemangiosarcoma. Evid Based Complement Alternat Med 2012;2012:384301
9. Ikekawa, T. 2001. Beneficial effects of mushrooms, edible and medicinal, on health care. International Journal of Medicinal Mushrooms 2001;3:291-298
10. Smith JE, Rowan NJ, Sullivan R. Medicinal Mushrooms: Their therapeutic properties and current medical usage with special emphasis on cancer treatments. Cancer Research UK. May 2002 (available online)
11. Kodama N, Komuta K, Nanba H. Can maitake MD-fraction aid cancer patients? Altern Med Rev 2002 Jun;7(3):236-9
12. Ajinimoto Company Information Publication. Lentinan: a new type of anticancer drug. Ajinimoto Co Inc 15-1 Kyobashi, Chuo-ku, Tokyo, Japan. 1984
13. On eating raw mushrooms. Retrieved from http://www.mykoweb.com/articles/EatingRawMushrooms.html
14. Nakazato H, Koike A, Saji S, Ogawa N, Sakamoto J. Efficacy of immunochemotherapy as adjuvant treatment after curative resection of gastric cancer. Study Group of Immunochemotherapy with PSK for Gastric Cancer. Lancet 1994 May 7;343(8906):1122-6
15. Wakui A, Kasai M, Konno K, Abe R, Kanamaru R, Takahashi K, Nakai Y, Yoshida Y, Koie H, Masuda H, et al. Randomized study of lentinan on patients with advanced gastric and colorectal cancer. Tohoku Lentinan Study Group. Gan To Kagaku Ryoho 1986 Apr;13(4 Pt 1):1050-9 (Article in Japanese but abstract in English)
16. Zhang M, Huang J, Xie X, Holman CD. Dietary intakes of mushrooms and green tea combine to reduce the risk of breast cancer in Chinese women. Int J Cancer 2009 Mar 15;124(6):1404-8
17. Shin A, Kim J, Lim SY, Kim G, Sung MK, Lee ES, Ro J. Dietary mushroom intake and the risk of breast cancer based on hormone receptor status. Nutr Cancer 2010;62(4):476-83
18. Lee SA, Kang D, Nishio H, Lee MJ, Kim DH, Han W, Yoo KY, Ahn SH, Choe KJ, Hirvonen A, Noh DY. Methylenetetrahydrofolate reductase polymorphism, diet, and breast cancer in Korean women. Exp Mol Med 2004 Apr 30;36(2):116-21
19. Hara M, Hanaoka T, Kobayashi M, Otani T, Adachi HY, Montani A, Natsukawa S, Shaura K, Koizumi Y, Kasuga Y, Matsuzawa T, Ikekawa T, Sasaki S, Tsugane S. Cruciferous vegetables, mushrooms, and gastrointestinal cancer risks in a multicenter, hospital-based case-control study in Japan. Nutr Cancer 2003;46(2):138-47
20. Ohwada S, Ikeya T, Yokomori T, Kusaba T, Roppongi T, Takahashi T, Nakamura S, Kakinuma S, Iwazaki S, Ishikawa H, Kawate S, Nakajima T, Morishita Y. Adjuvant immunochemotherapy with oral Tegafur/Uracil plus PSK in patients with stage II or III colorectal cancer: a randomised controlled study. Br J Cancer 2004 Mar 8;90(5):1003-10

21. Xu T, Beelman RB, Lambert JD. The cancer preventive effects of edible mushrooms. Anticancer Agents Med Chem 2012 Dec;12(10):1255-63
22. Deng G, Lin H, Seidman A, Fornier M, D'Andrea G, Wesa K, Yeung S, Cunningham-Rundles S, Vickers AJ, Cassileth B. A phase I/II trial of a polysaccharide extract from Grifola frondosa (Maitake mushroom) in breast cancer patients: immunological effects. J Cancer Res Clin Oncol 2009 Sep;135(9):1215-21
23. Luk SU, Lee TK, Liu J, Lee DT, Chiu YT, Ma S, Ng IO, Wong YC, Chan FL, Ling MT. Chemopreventive effect of PSP through targeting of prostate cancer stem cell-like population. PLoS One 2011;6(5):e19804

References for Chapters 8 and 27: Resveratrol

1. Aggarwal BB, Bhardwaj A, Aggarwal RS, Seeram NP, Shishodia S, Takada Y. Role of resveratrol in prevention and therapy of cancer: preclinical and clinical studies. Anticancer Res 2004 Sep-Oct;24(5A):2783-840
2. Betz J. Resveratrol and its Effects on Human Health and Longevity - Myth or Miracle? Truth Publishing International Ltd Taiwan 2011 (available online)
3. Resveratrol. Retrieved from http://en.wikipedia.org/wiki/Resveratrol
4. Memorial Sloan Kettering Cancer Centre: About herbs, botanicals, and other products. http://www.mskcc.org/cancer-care/herb/resveratrol
5. Lin HY, Tang HY, Davis FB, Davis PJ. Resveratrol and apoptosis. Ann N Y Acad Sci 2011 Jan;1215:79-88
6. Shukla Y, Singh R. Resveratrol and cellular mechanisms of cancer prevention. Ann N Y Acad Sci 2011 Jan;1215:1-8
7. Gupta SC, Kannappan R, Reuter S, Kim JH, Aggarwal BB. Chemosensitization of tumors by resveratrol. Ann N Y Acad Sci 2011 Jan;1215:150-60
8. Patel KR, Scott E, Brown VA, Gescher AJ, Steward WP, Brown K. Clinical trials of resveratrol. Ann N Y Acad Sci 2011 Jan;1215:161-9
9. Schoonen WM, Salinas CA, Kiemeney LA, Stanford JL. Alcohol consumption and risk of prostate cancer in middle-aged men. Int J Cancer 2005 Jan 1;113(1):133-40
10. Chao C, Haque R, Van Den Eeden SK, Caan BJ, Poon KY, Quinn VP. Red wine consumption and risk of prostate cancer: the California men's health study. Int J Cancer 2010 Jan 1;126(1):171-9
11. Sutcliffe S, Giovannucci E, Leitzmann MF, Rimm EB, Stampfer MJ, Willett WC, Platz EA. A prospective cohort study of red wine consumption and risk of prostate cancer. Int J Cancer 2007 Apr 1;120(7):1529-35
12. Resveratrol (Linus Pauling Institute) Retrieved from http://lpi.oregonstate.edu/infocenter/phytochemicals/resveratrol/
13. National Cancer Institute Factsheet on Red Wine and Cancer Prevention http://www.cancer.gov/cancertopics/factsheet/prevention/redwine
14. Magee JB, Smith BJ, Romando A. Resveratrol content of Muscadine berries is affected by disease control spray program. Hort Science 2002;37(2):358-361

15. Smith BJ. Fruit Quality, Phytochemical Content, and Disease Severity of Muscadine Grapes Affected by Fungicide Applications. Pharmaceutical Crops 2013;4:21-37
16. Prof Karen Brown of University of Leicester, audio clip on-http://www2.le.ac.uk/offices/press/press-releases/2012/december/new-evidence-on-how-compound-found-in-red-wine-can-help-prevent-cancer
17. Jang M, Cai L, Udeani GO, Slowing KV, Thomas CF, Beecher CW, Fong HH, Farnsworth NR, Kinghorn AD, Mehta RG, Moon RC, Pezzuto JM. Cancer chemopreventive activity of resveratrol, a natural product derived from grapes. Science 1997 Jan 10;275(5297):218-20
18. Thick-skinned red grapes, etc, retrieved from http://www.examiner.com/article/thick-skinned-red-grapes-and-the-wines-they-produce-show-major-health-benefits
19. Bartender, a glass of medicine please. Retrieved from http://www.winespectator.com/webfeature/show/id/Bartender-a-Glass-of-Medicine-Please_4545
20. Friedlander Jr., Blaine P. Higher levels of resveratrol found among N.Y. red wines. Cornell Chronicle.Web. 29.20 (5 Feb 1998). Ithaca, NY, USA: Cornell University. www.news.cornell.edu/Chronicle/98/2.5.98/resveratrol.html.
21. Cantos E, Espín JC, Tomás-Barberán FA. Postharvest induction modeling method using UV irradiation pulses for obtaining resveratrol-enriched table grapes: a new "functional" fruit? J Agric Food Chem 2001 Oct;49(10):5052-8
22. Szekeres T, Saiko P, Fritzer-Szekeres M, Djavan B, Jäger W. Chemopreventive effects of resveratrol and resveratrol derivatives. Ann N Y Acad Sci 2011 Jan;1215:89-95
23. Walle T. Bioavailability of resveratrol. Ann N Y Acad Sci 2011 Jan;1215:9-15
24. Delmas D, Aires V, Limagne E, Dutartre P, Mazué F, Ghiringhelli F, Latruffe N. Transport, stability, and biological activity of resveratrol. Ann N Y Acad Sci 2011 Jan;1215:48-59
25. Prof Karen Brown of University of Leicester, audio clip on- http://www.nutraingredients-usa.com/Research/Re-forming-resveratrol-Bioavailability-issues-are-no-more-as-researchers-reveal-metabolites-regenerate?utm_source=copyright&utm_medium=OnSite&utm_campaign=copyright
26. Patel KR, Brown VA, Jones DJ, Britton RG, Hemingway D, Miller AS, West KP, Booth TD, Perloff M, Crowell JA, Brenner DE, Steward WP, Gescher AJ, Brown K. Clinical pharmacology of resveratrol and its metabolites in colorectal cancer patients. Cancer Res 2010 Oct 1;70(19):7392-9
27. Building a better resveratrol, etc. Retrieved from http://www.resveratrol-news.com/building-a-better-resveratrol-is-it-time-to-switch-from-resveratrol-to-pterostilbene/101/

References for Chapters 9 and 28: Selenium (and Magnesium)

1. Drake EN. 2001. Selenium: Are you getting enough to reduce your risk of cancer? Writer's Showcase

2. Shamberger RJ, Tytko SA, Willis CE. Antioxidants and cancer. Part VI. Selenium and age-adjusted human cancer mortality. Arch Environ Health 1976 Sep-Oct;31(5):231-5
3. Salonen JT, Alfthan G, Huttunen JK, Puska P. Association between serum selenium and the risk of cancer. Am J Epidemiol 1984 Sep;120(3):342-9
4. Schrauzer GN, Ishmael D. Effects of selenium and of arsenic on the genesis of spontaneous mammary tumors in inbred C3H mice. Ann Clin Lab Sci 1974 Nov-Dec;4(6):441-7
5. Watrach AM, Milner JA, Watrach MA, Poirier KA. Inhibition of human breast cancer cells by selenium. Cancer Lett 1984 Nov;25(1):41-7
6. Clark LC, Combs GF Jr, Turnbull BW, Slate EH, Chalker DK, Chow J, Davis LS, Glover RA, Graham GF, Gross EG, Krongrad A, Lesher JL Jr, Park HK, Sanders BB Jr, Smith CL, Taylor JR. Effects of selenium supplementation for cancer prevention in patients with carcinoma of the skin. A randomized controlled trial. Nutritional Prevention of Cancer Study Group. JAMA 1996 Dec 25;276(24):1957-63
7. Yu SY, Zhu YJ, LI WG, Huang QS, Huang CZ, Zhang QN, Hou C. A preliminary report on the intervention trials of primary liver cancer in high-risk populations with nutritional supplementation of selenium in China. Biol Trace Elem Res 1991 Jun;29(3):289-94
8. Blot WJ, LI JY, Taylor PR, Guo W, Dawsey S, Wang GQ, Yang CS, Zheng SF, Gail M, LI GY, et al. Nutrition intervention trials in Linxian, China: supplementation with specific vitamin/mineral combinations, cancer incidence, and disease-specific mortality in the general population. J Natl Cancer Inst 1993 Sep 15;85(18):1483-92
9. LI JY, Taylor PR, LI B, Dawsey S, Wang GQ, Ershow AG, Guo W, Liu SF, Yang CS, Shen Q, et al. Nutrition intervention trials in Linxian, China: multiple vitamin/mineral supplementation, cancer incidence, and disease-specific mortality among adults with esophageal dysplasia. J Natl Cancer Inst 1993 Sep 15;85(18):1492-8
10. Klein EA, Thompson IM Jr, Tangen CM, Crowley JJ, Lucia MS, Goodman PJ, Minasian LM, Ford LG, Parnes HL, Gaziano JM, Karp DD, Lieber MM, Walther PJ, Klotz L, Parsons JK, Chin JL, Darke AK, Lippman SM, Goodman GE, Meyskens FL Jr, Baker LH. Vitamin E and the risk of prostate cancer: the Selenium and Vitamin E Cancer Prevention Trial (SELECT). JAMA 2011 Oct 12;306(14):1549-56
11. Thomson CD, Chisholm A, McLachlan SK, Campbell JM. Brazil nuts: an effective way to improve selenium status. Am J Clin Nutr 2008 Feb;87(2):379-84
12. Brazil nuts and variation in selenium content. 2012. Retrieved from http://honey-guide.com/2012/11/19/brazil-nuts-and-selenium/
13. Longnecker MP, Taylor PR, Levander OA, Howe M, Veillon C, McAdam PA, Patterson KY, Holden JM, Stampfer MJ, Morris JS, et al. Selenium in diet, blood, and toenails in relation to human health in a seleniferous area. Am J Clin Nutr 1991 May;53(5):1288-94
14. Tinggi U. Essentiality and toxicity of selenium and its status in Australia: a review. Toxicol Lett 2003 Jan 31;137(1-2):103-10

15. Folsom AR, Hong CP. Magnesium intake and reduced risk of colon cancer in a prospective study of women. Am J Epidemiol 2006 Feb 1;163(3):232-5
16. Larsson SC, Bergkvist L, Wolk A. Magnesium intake in relation to risk of colorectal cancer in women. JAMA 2005 Jan 5;293(1):86-9
17. Qu X, Jin F, Hao Y, Zhu Z, LI H, Tang T, Dai K. Nonlinear association between magnesium intake and the risk of colorectal cancer. Eur J Gastroenterol Hepatol 2013 Mar;25(3):309-18
18. Wark PA, Lau R, Norat T, Kampman E. Magnesium intake and colorectal tumor risk: a case-control study and meta-analysis. Am J Clin Nutr 2012 Sep;96(3):622-31
19. Magnesium and cancer. Retrieved from http://www.mgwater.com/rod02.shtml
20. Sinha R, Said TK, Medina D. Organic and inorganic selenium compounds inhibit mouse mammary cell growth in vitro by different cellular pathways. Cancer Lett 1996 Oct 22;107(2):277-84
21. Sinha R, Kiley SC, Lu JX, Thompson HJ, Moraes R, Jaken S, Medina D. Effects of methylselenocysteine on PKC activity, cdk2 phosphorylation and gadd gene expression in synchronized mouse mammary epithelial tumor cells. Cancer Lett 1999 Nov 15;146(2):135-45
22. Kiremidjian-Schumacher L, Roy M, Wishe HI, Cohen MW, Stotzky G. Supplementation with selenium and human immune cell functions. II. Effect on cytotoxic lymphocytes and natural killer cells. Biol Trace Elem Res 1994 Apr-May;41(1-2):115-27
23. Kiremidjian-Schumacher L, Roy M, Wishe HI, Cohen MW, Stotzky G. Regulation of cellular immune responses by selenium. Biol Trace Elem Res 1992 Apr-Jun;33:23-35
24. Peretz A, Nève J, Desmedt J, Duchateau J, Dramaix M, Famaey JP. Lymphocyte response is enhanced by supplementation of elderly subjects with selenium-enriched yeast. Am J Clin Nutr 1991 May;53(5):1323-8
25. Hercberg S, Galan P, Preziosi P, Bertrais S, Mennen L, Malvy D, Roussel AM, Favier A, Briançon S. The SU.VI.MAX Study: a randomized, placebo-controlled trial of the health effects of antioxidant vitamins and minerals. Arch Intern Med 2004 Nov 22;164(21):2335-42
26. Ip C. Lessons from basic research in selenium and cancer prevention. J Nutr 1998 Nov;128(11):1845-54
27. Ohta Y, Kobayashi Y, Konishi S, Hirano S. Speciation analysis of selenium metabolites in urine and breath by HPLC- and GC-inductively coupled plasma-MS after administration of selenomethionine and methylselenocysteine to rats. Chem Res Toxicol 2009 Nov;22(11):1795-801

References for Chapters 10 and 29: Carrots, Carotene and Colour

1. Mignone LI, Giovannucci E, Newcomb PA, Titus-Ernstoff L, Trentham-Dietz A, Hampton JM, Willett WC, Egan KM. Dietary carotenoids and the risk of invasive breast cancer. Int J Cancer 2009 Jun 15;124(12):2929-37

2. Boggs DA, Palmer JR, Wise LA, Spiegelman D, Stampfer MJ, Adams-Campbell LL, Rosenberg L. Fruit and vegetable intake in relation to risk of breast cancer in the Black Women's Health Study. Am J Epidemiol 2010 Dec 1;172(11):1268-79
3. Chen L, Stacewicz-Sapuntzakis M, Duncan C, Sharifi R, Ghosh L, van Breemen R, Ashton D, Bowen PE. Oxidative DNA damage in prostate cancer patients consuming tomato sauce-based entrees as a whole-food intervention. J Natl Cancer Inst 2001 Dec 19;93(24):1872-9
4. Giovannucci E, Liu Y, Platz EA, Stampfer MJ, Willett WC. Risk factors for prostate cancer incidence and progression in the health professionals follow-up study. Int J Cancer 2007 Oct 1;121(7):1571-8
5. Ferenczi A. Tumor Treatment with Red Beets and Anthocyans, respectively. Zeitschrift fuer die gesamte innere Medizin und ihre Grenzgebiete, VEB Georg Thieme Verlag, Leipzig, Bd. 16, 1961, 180
6. Büchner FL, Bueno-de-Mesquita HB, Ros MM, Overvad K, Dahm CC, Hansen L, Tjønneland A, et al. Variety in fruit and vegetable consumption and the risk of lung cancer in the European prospective investigation into cancer and nutrition. Cancer Epidemiol Biomarkers Prev 2010 Sep;19(9):2278-86
7. Farneti B, Schouten RE, Woltering EJ. Low temperature-induced lycopene degradation in red ripe tomato evaluated by remittance spectroscopy. Postharvest Biology and Technology 2012 Nov;73:22-27
8. van het Hof KH, de Boer BC, Tijburg LB, Lucius BR, Zijp I, West CE, Hautvast JG, Weststrate JA. Carotenoid bioavailability in humans from tomatoes processed in different ways determined from the carotenoid response in the triglyceride-rich lipoprotein fraction of plasma after a single consumption and in plasma after four days of consumption. J Nutr 2000 May;130(5):1189-96
9. Fielding JM, Rowley KG, Cooper P, O'Dea K. Increases in plasma lycopene concentration after consumption of tomatoes cooked with olive oil. Asia Pac J Clin Nutr 2005;14(2):131-6
10. Unlu NZ, Bohn T, Clinton SK, Schwartz SJ. Carotenoid absorption from salad and salsa by humans is enhanced by the addition of avocado or avocado oil. J Nutr 2005 Mar;135(3):431-6
11. Carrots, nutrition and good health. Retrieved from http://www.carrotmuseum.co.uk/nutrition.html#general
12. Zhang D, Hamauzu Y. Phenolic compounds and their antioxidant properties in different tissues of carrots (*Daucus carota* L.) J Food Agric Environ 2004;2:95–100
13. Astley SB, Elliott RM, Archer DB, Southon S. Evidence that dietary supplementation with carotenoids and carotenoid-rich foods modulates the DNA damage: repair balance in human lymphocytes. Br J Nutr 2004 Jan;91(1):63-72
14. Clarke N, Germain P, Altucci L, Gronemeyer H. Retinoids: potential in cancer prevention and therapy. Expert Rev Mol Med 2004 Nov 30;6(25):1-23
15. Oldridge EE, Walker HF, Stower MJ, Simms MS, Mann VM, Collins AT, Pellacani D, Maitland NJ. Retinoic acid represses invasion and stem cell

phenotype by induction of the metastasis suppressors RARRES1 and LXN. Oncogenesis 2013 Apr 15;2:e45

16. Could carrots beat prostate cancer? Retrieved from http://www.dailymail.co.uk/health/article-2310143/Could-effective-battle-prostate-cancer-according-scientists.html
17. Hughes DA, Wright AJ, Finglas PM, Peerless AC, Bailey AL, Astley SB, Pinder AC, Southon S. The effect of beta-carotene supplementation on the immune function of blood monocytes from healthy male nonsmokers. J Lab Clin Med 1997 Mar;129(3):309-17
18. Nahum A, Zeller L, Danilenko M, Prall OW, Watts CK, Sutherland RL, Levy J, Sharoni Y. Lycopene inhibition of IGF-induced cancer cell growth depends on the level of cyclin D1. Eur J Nutr 2006 Aug;45(5):275-82
19. Huang CS, Liao JW, Hu ML. Lycopene inhibits experimental metastasis of human hepatoma SK-Hep-1 cells in athymic nude mice. J Nutr 2008 Mar;138(3):538-43
20. Stahl W, Sies H. Carotenoids and flavonoids contribute to nutritional protection against skin damage from sunlight. Mol Biotechnol 2007 Sep;37(1):26-30
21. Kobaek-Larsen M, Christensen LP, Vach W, Ritskes-Hoitinga J, Brandt K. Inhibitory effects of feeding with carrots or (-)-falcarinol on development of azoxymethane-induced preneoplastic lesions in the rat colon. J Agric Food Chem 2005 Mar 9;53(5):1823-7
22. Raw carrots help prevent colon cancer, say Danish researchers. Retrieved from http://www.timeshighereducation.co.uk/193975.article
23. Holick CN, Michaud DS, Stolzenberg-Solomon R, Mayne ST, Pietinen P, Taylor PR, Virtamo J, Albanes D. Dietary carotenoids, serum beta-carotene, and retinol and risk of lung cancer in the alpha-tocopherol, beta-carotene cohort study. Am J Epidemiol 2002 Sep 15;156(6):536-47
24. Satia JA, Littman A, Slatore CG, Galanko JA, White E. Long-term use of beta-carotene, retinol, lycopene, and lutein supplements and lung cancer risk: results from the VITamins And Lifestyle (VITAL) study. Am J Epidemiol 2009 Apr 1;169(7):815-28
25. Beta-carotene and cancer risk. Position statement Cancer Council Australia. Retrieved from http://www.cancer.org.au/content/pdf/CancerControlPolicy/PositionStatements/PS_Betacarotene_and_cancer_risk_September_2009.pdf
26. International Agency for Research on Cancer. Carotenoids. Lyon: IARC. 1998. Retrieved from http://www.iarc.fr/en/publications/pdfs-online/prev/handbook2/Handbook2_Carotenoids.pdf

References for Chapters 11 and 30: Probiotics

1. Velicer CM, Heckbert SR, Lampe JW, Potter JD, Robertson CA, Taplin SH. Antibiotic use in relation to the risk of breast cancer. JAMA 2004 Feb 18;291(7):827-35

2. Morrier JJ, Suchett-Kaye G, Nguyen D, Rocca JP, Blanc-Benon J, Barsotti O. Antimicrobial activity of amalgams, alloys and their elements and phases. Dent Mater 1998 Mar;14(2):150-7
3. Summers AO, Wireman J, Vimy MJ, Lorscheider FL, Marshall B, Levy SB, Bennett S, Billard L. Mercury released from dental "silver" fillings provokes an increase in mercury- and antibiotic-resistant bacteria in oral and intestinal floras of primates. Antimicrob Agents Chemother 1993 Apr;37(4):825-34
4. Euler, L. Still taking a probiotic supplement? Five reasons to consider ditching it. Retrieved from www.cancerdefeated.com/still-taking-a-probiotic-supplement-5-reasons-to-consider-ditching-it-2/1271/
5. Moshfegh AJ, Friday JE, Goldman JP, Ahuja JK. Presence of inulin and oligofructose in the diets of Americans. J Nutr 1999 Jul;129(7 Suppl):1407S-11S
6. Aso Y, Akaza H, Kotake T, Tsukamoto T, Imai K, Naito S. Preventive effect of a Lactobacillus casei preparation on the recurrence of superficial bladder cancer in a double-blind trial. The BLP Study Group. Eur Urol 1995;27(2):104-9
7. Hayatsu H, Hayatsu T. Suppressing effect of Lactobacillus casei administration on the urinary mutagenicity arising from ingestion of fried ground beef in the human. Cancer Lett 1993 Sep 30;73(2-3):173-9
8. Goldin BR, Gorbach SL. Effect of Lactobacillus acidophilus dietary supplements on 1,2-dimethylhydrazine dihydrochloride-induced intestinal cancer in rats. J Natl Cancer Inst 1980 Feb;64(2):263-5
9. Ishikawa H, Akedo I, Otani T, Suzuki T, Nakamura T, Takeyama I, Ishiguro S, Miyaoka E, Sobue T, Kakizoe T. Randomized trial of dietary fiber and Lactobacillus casei administration for prevention of colorectal tumors. Int J Cancer 2005 Sep 20;116(5):762-7
10. Rafter J, Bennett M, Caderni G, Clune Y et al.Dietary synbiotics reduce cancer risk factors in polypectomized and colon cancer patients. Am J Clin Nutr 2007 Feb;85(2):488-96
11. Malhotra SL. Dietary factors in a study of cancer colon from Cancer Registry, with special reference to the role of saliva, milk and fermented milk products and vegetable fibre. Med Hypotheses 1977 May-Jun;3(3):122-6
12. Peters RK, Pike MC, Garabrant D, Mack TM. Diet and colon cancer in Los Angeles County, California. Cancer Causes Control 1992 Sep;3(5):457-73
13. Young TB, Wolf DA Case-control study of proximal and distal colon cancer and diet in Wisconsin. Int J Cancer 1988 Aug 15;42(2):167-75
14. Lê MG, Moulton LH, Hill C, Kramar A. Consumption of dairy produce and alcohol in a case-control study of breast cancer. J Natl Cancer Inst 1986 Sep;77(3):633-6
15. van't Veer P, Dekker JM, Lamers JW, Kok FJ, Schouten EG, Brants HA, Sturmans F, Hermus RJ. Consumption of fermented milk products and breast cancer: a case-control study in The Netherlands. Cancer Res 1989 Jul 15;49(14):4020-3

16. Kumar M, Kumar A, Nagpal R, Mohania D, Behare P, Verma V, Kumar P, Poddar D, Aggarwal PK, Henry CJ, Jain S, Yadav H. Cancer-preventing attributes of probiotics: an update. Int J Food Sci Nutr 2010 Aug;61(5):473-96
17. Kahouli I, Tomaro-Duchesneau C, Prakash S. Probiotics in colorectal cancer (CRC) with emphasis on mechanisms of actions and current prospectives. J Med Microbiol 2013 Aug;62(Pt 8):1107-23
18. Rafter J. The effects of probiotics on colon cancer development. Nutr Res Rev 2004 Dec;17(2):277-84
19. Pool-Zobel BL, Sauer J. Overview of experimental data on reduction of colorectal cancer risk by inulin-type fructans. J Nutr 2007 Nov;137(11 Suppl):2580S-2584S
20. Uccello M, Malaguarnera G, Basile F, D'agata V, Malaguarnera M, Bertino G, Vacante M, Drago F, Biondi A. Potential role of probiotics on colorectal cancer prevention. BMC Surg 2012;12 Suppl 1:S35
21. Wollowski I, Rechkemmer G, Pool-Zobel BL. Protective role of probiotics and prebiotics in colon cancer. Am J Clin Nutr 2001 Feb;73(2 Suppl):451S-455S
22. Greenhill C. Gut microbiota: Anti-cancer therapies affected by gut microbiota. Nat Rev Gastroenterol Hepatol 2014 Jan;11(1):1

References for Chapter 12: Fibre

1. Murphy N, Norat T, Ferrari P, Jenab M, Bueno-de-Mesquita B, Skeie G et al. Dietary fibre intake and risks of cancers of the colon and rectum in the European prospective investigation into cancer and nutrition (EPIC). PLoS One 2012;7(6):e39361
2. Lu R, Wang X, Sun DF, Tian XQ, Zhao SL, Chen YX, Fang JY. Folic acid and sodium butyrate prevent tumorigenesis in a mouse model of colorectal cancer. Epigenetics 2008 Nov;3(6):330-5
3. D'Argenio G, Cosenza V, Delle Cave M, Iovino P, Delle Valle N, Lombardi G, Mazzacca G. Butyrate enemas in experimental colitis and protection against large bowel cancer in a rat model. Gastroenterology 1996 Jun;110(6):1727-34
4. Chen HM, Yu YN, Wang JL, Lin YW, Kong X, Yang CQ et al. Decreased dietary fiber intake and structural alteration of gut microbiota in patients with advanced colorectal adenoma. Am J Clin Nutr 2013 May;97(5):1044-52
5. Jiang B, Zhang X, Du LL, Wang Y, Liu DB, Han CZ, Jing JX, Zhao XW, Xu XQ. Possible roles of insulin, IGF-1 and IGFBPs in initiation and progression of colorectal cancer. World J Gastroenterol 2014 Feb 14;20(6):1608-13
6. Sandhu MS, Dunger DB, Giovannucci EL. Insulin, insulin-like growth factor-I (IGF-I), IGF binding proteins, their biologic interactions, and colorectal cancer. J Natl Cancer Inst 2002 Jul 3;94(13):972-80
7. Petrakis NL, King EB. Cytological abnormalities in nipple aspirates of breast fluid from women with severe constipation. Lancet 1981 Nov 28;2(8257):1203-4

8. Vitanzo PC Jr, Hong ES. Does a high-fiber dietary supplement of wheat bran reduce the recurrence rate of colorectal adenomas? J Fam Pract 2000 Jul;49(7):656
9. Bonithon-Kopp C, Kronborg O, Giacosa A, Räth U, Faivre J. Calcium and fibre supplementation in prevention of colorectal adenoma recurrence: a randomised intervention trial. European Cancer Prevention Organisation Study Group. Lancet 2000 Oct 14;356(9238):1300-6

References for Chapter 13 and 31: Iodine

1. Brownstein D. 2004. Iodine: Why you need it, Why you can't live without it. Medical Alternative Press, Michigan
2. Derry DM. 2001. Breast cancer and iodine. Trafford, Canada.
3. Hardefeldt PJ, Eslick GD, Edirimanne S. Benign thyroid disease is associated with breast cancer: a meta-analysis. Breast Cancer Res Treat 2012 Jun;133(3):1169-77
4. Turken O, NarIn Y, DemIrbas S, Onde ME, Sayan O, KandemIr EG, Yaylaci M, Ozturk A. Breast cancer in association with thyroid disorders. Breast Cancer Res 2003;5(5):R110-3
5. Cann SA, van Netten JP, van Netten C. Hypothesis: iodine, selenium and the development of breast cancer. Cancer Causes Control 2000 Feb;11(2):121-7
6. Serra Majem LL, Tresserras R, Canela J, Salleras L. Dietary iodine deficiency and breast cancer mortality: an ecological study. Int J Epidemiol 1988;17:686-687
7. Kato N, Funahashi H, Ando K, Takagi H. Suppressive effect of iodine preparations on proliferation of DMBA-induced breast cancer in rat. J Jpn Soc Cancer Ther 1994;29:582-588
8. Stoddard FR 2nd, Brooks AD, Eskin BA, Johannes GJ Iodine alters gene expression in the MCF7 breast cancer cell line: evidence for an anti-estrogen effect of iodine. Int J Med Sci 2008 Jul 8;5(4):189-96
9. Soriano O, Delgado G, Anguiano B, Petrosyan P, Molina-Servín ED, Gonsebatt ME, Aceves C. Antineoplastic effect of iodine and iodide in dimethylbenz[a]anthracene-induced mammary tumors: association between lactoperoxidase and estrogen-adduct production. Endocr Relat Cancer 2011 Jul 25;18(4):529-39
10. Funahashi H, Imai T, Mase T, Sekiya M, Yokoi K, Hayashi Het al. Seaweed prevents breast cancer? Jpn J Cancer Res 2001 May;92(5):483-7
11. Krouse TB, Eskin BA, Mobini J. Age-related changes resembling fibrocystic disease in iodine-blocked rat breasts. Arch Pathol Lab Med 1979 Nov;103(12):631-4
12. Kessler JH. The effect of supraphysiologic levels of iodine on patients with cyclic mastalgia. Breast J 2004 Jul-Aug;10(4):328-36
13. Bezpalov VG, Barash NIu, Ivanova OA, Semënov II, Aleksandrov VA, Semiglazov VF. Investigation of the drug "Mamoclam" for the treatment of patients with fibroadenomatosis of the breast (Article in Russian). Vopr Onkol 2005;51(2):236-41

14. Hartmann LC, Sellers TA, Frost MH, Lingle WL, Degnim AC, Ghosh K, Vierkant RA, et al. Benign breast disease and the risk of breast cancer. N Engl J Med 2005 Jul 21;353(3):229-37
15. Smyth PP. The thyroid, iodine and breast cancer. Breast Cancer Res 2003;5(5):235-8
16. Arroyo-Helguera O, Rojas E, Delgado G, Aceves C. Signaling pathways involved in the antiproliferative effect of molecular iodine in normal and tumoral breast cells: evidence that 6-iodolactone mediates apoptotic effects. Endocr Relat Cancer 2008 Dec;15(4):1003-11
17. Venturi S. Is there a role for iodine in breast diseases? The Breast 2001 Oct;10(5):379-82
18. Funahashi H, Imai T, Tanaka Y, Tobinaga J, Wada M, Morita T, Yamada F et al. Suppressive effect of iodine on DMBA-induced breast tumor growth in the rat. J Surg Oncol 1996 Mar;61(3):209-13
19. Kogai T, Taki K, Brent GA. Enhancement of sodium/iodide symporter expression in thyroid and breast cancer. Endocr Relat Cancer 2006 Sep;13(3):797-826
20. Gérard AC, Humblet K, Wilvers C, Poncin S, Derradji H et al. Iodine-deficiency-induced long lasting angiogenic reaction in thyroid cancers occurs via a vascular endothelial growth factor-hypoxia inducible factor-1-dependent, but not a reactive oxygen species-dependent, pathway. Thyroid 2012 Jul;22(7):699-708

References for Chapter 14: Everyday superfoods

1. Boyer J, Liu RH. Apple phytochemicals and their health benefits. Nutr J 2004 May 12;3:5
2. Gerhauser C. Cancer chemopreventive potential of apples, apple juice, and apple components. Planta Med 2008 Oct;74(13):1608-24
3. Sun J, Liu RH. Apple phytochemical extracts inhibit proliferation of estrogen-dependent and estrogen-independent human breast cancer cells through cell cycle modulation. J Agric Food Chem 2008 Dec 24;56(24):11661-7
4. Reagan-Shaw S, Eggert D, Mukhtar H, Ahmad N. Antiproliferative effects of apple peel extract against cancer cells. Nutr Cancer 2010;62(4):517-24
5. Liu JR, Dong HW, Chen BQ, Zhao P, Liu RH. Fresh apples suppress mammary carcinogenesis and proliferative activity and induce apoptosis in mammary tumors of the Sprague-Dawley rat. J Agric Food Chem 2009 Jan 14;57(1):297-304
6. Lang SS. In flurry of studies, researcher details role of apples in inhibiting breast cancer. Cornell Chronicle (Cornell University) retrieved from http://www.news.cornell.edu/stories/2009/02/liu-details-role-apples-inhibiting-breast-cancer
7. Miller JA, Lang JE, Ley M, Nagle R, Hsu CH, Thompson PA, Cordova C, Waer A, Chow HH. Human breast tissue disposition and bioactivity of limonene in women with early-stage breast cancer. Cancer Prev Res (Phila) 2013 Jun;6(6):577-84

8. Monroe KR, Murphy SP, Kolonel LN, Pike MC. Prospective study of grapefruit intake and risk of breast cancer in postmenopausal women: the Multiethnic Cohort Study. Br J Cancer 2007 Aug 6;97(3):440-5
9. Baghurst K (CSIRO). The health benefits of citrus fruits. Published by Horticulture Australia Ltd 2003 (available online)
10. Song JK, Bae JM. Citrus fruit intake and breast cancer risk: a quantitative systematic review. J Breast Cancer 2013 Mar;16(1):72-6
11. Evers E. Citrus fruit significantly reduces breast cancer risk in latest systematic review. Retrieved from http://www.naturalnews.com/040193_breast_cancer_prevention_foods_citrus_fruit.html#ixzz2SP2y2X8J

References for Chapter 15: What you can do without

1. Baade PD, Meng X, Sinclair C, Youl P. Estimating the future burden of cancers preventable by better diet and physical activity in Australia. Med J Aust 2012 Mar 19;196(5):337-40
2. Chen WY, Rosner B, Hankinson SE, Colditz GA, Willett WC. Moderate alcohol consumption during adult life, drinking patterns, and breast cancer risk. JAMA 2011 Nov 2;306(17):1884-90
3. Pan A, Sun Q, Bernstein AM, Schulze MB, Manson JE, Stampfer MJ, Willett WC, Hu FB. Red meat consumption and mortality: results from 2 prospective cohort studies. Arch Intern Med 2012 Apr 9;172(7):555-63
4. Liu CY, Hsu YH, Wu MT, Pan PC, Ho CK, Su L, Xu X, LI Y, Christiani DC; Kaohsiung Leukemia Research Group. Cured meat, vegetables, and bean-curd foods in relation to childhood acute leukemia risk: a population based case-control study. BMC Cancer 2009 Jan 13;9:15
5. Rogers IS, Northstone K, Dunger DB, Cooper AR, Ness AR, Emmett PM. Diet throughout childhood and age at menarche in a contemporary cohort of British girls. Public Health Nutr 2010 Dec;13(12):2052-63
6. Lustig R. Sugar: The bitter truth. Retrieved from https://www.youtube.com/watch?v=dBnniua6-oM
7. Gillespie D. Sweet Poison: Why Sugar is Making Us Fat. Viking Australia 2008
8. Ho VW, Leung K, Hsu A, Luk B, Lai J, Shen SY, Minchinton AI, Waterhouse D, Bally MB, Lin W, Nelson BH, Sly LM, Krystal G. A low carbohydrate, high protein diet slows tumor growth and prevents cancer initiation. Cancer Res 2011 Jul 1;71(13):4484-93
9. Augustin LS, Dal Maso L, La Vecchia C, Parpinel M, Negri E, Vaccarella S, Kendall CW, Jenkins DJ, Francesch S. Dietary glycemic index and glycemic load, and breast cancer risk: a case-control study. Ann Oncol 2001 Nov;12(11):1533-8
10. Augustin LS, Polesel J, Bosetti C, Kendall CW, La Vecchia C, Parpinel M, Conti E, Montella M, Franceschi S, Jenkins DJ, Dal Maso L. Dietary glycemic index, glycemic load and ovarian cancer risk: a case-control study in Italy. Ann Oncol 2003 Jan;14(1):78-84

11. Franceschi S, Dal Maso L, Augustin L, Negri E, Parpinel M, Boyle P, Jenkins DJ, La Vecchia C. Dietary glycemic load and colorectal cancer risk. Ann Oncol 2001 Feb;12(2):173-8
12. Randi G, Ferraroni M, Talamini R, Garavello W, Deandrea S, Decarli A, Franceschi S, La Vecchia C. Glycemic index, glycemic load and thyroid cancer risk. Ann Oncol 2008 Feb;19(2):380-3
13. LI C, Balluz LS, Ford ES, Okoro CA, Tsai J, Zhao G. Association between diagnosed diabetes and self-reported cancer among U.S. adults: findings from the 2009 Behavioral Risk Factor Surveillance System. Diabetes Care 2011 Jun;34(6):1365-8
14. Yu H, Rohan T. Role of insulin-like growth factor family in cancer development and progression. J Natl Cancer Inst 2000; 92:1472-1489
15. Hankinson SE, Willett WC, Colditz GA, Hunter DJ, Michaud DS, Deroo B, Rosner B, Speizer FE, Pollak M. Circulating concentrations of insulin-like growth factor-I and risk of breast cancer. Lancet 1998 May 9;351(9113):1393-6
16. Manousos O, Souglakos J, Bosetti C et al. IGF-1 and IGF-II in relation to colorectal cancer. Int J Cancer 1999; 83:15-7
17. Greenfield JR, McCormack AI. Medication to prevent breast cancer - too much to swallow? Med J Aust 2012 Mar 19;196(5):314
18. Ligibel J. Obesity and breast cancer. Oncology (Williston Park) 2011 Oct;25(11):994-1000
19. Protani M, Coory M, Martin JH. Effect of obesity on survival of women with breast cancer: systematic review and meta-analysis. Breast Cancer Res Treat 2010;123:627-35
20. Chlebowski RT. The obesity and breast cancer connection: advancing the agenda. Oncology (Williston Park) 2011 Oct;25(11):1007, 1011-2
21. What You Need To Know About Obesity and Cancer. Retrieved from http://www.aicr.org/learn-more-about-cancer/infographic-obesity-and-cancer.html
22. Campbell TC, Campbell TM. The China Study. Benbella Books, Texas. 2006
23. Plant J. Your Life in Your Hands. Virgin Books Ltd, London. 2007
24. Petersen IB. The Maasai keep healthy despite a high-fat diet. Retrieved from http://sciencenordic.com/maasai-keep-healthy-despite-high-fat-diet

References for Chapter 16: How to eat

1. Viegas O, Amaro LF, Ferreira IM, Pinho O. Inhibitory effect of antioxidant-rich marinades on the formation of heterocyclic aromatic amines in pan-fried beef. J Agric Food Chem 2012 Jun 20;60(24):6235-40
2. Schardt D. Microwave myths. Retrieved from http://www.cspinet.org/nah/04_05/microwavemyths.pdf
3. Verkerk R, Dekker M. Glucosinolates and myrosinase activity in red cabbage (Brassica oleracea L. var. Capitata f. rubra DC.) after various microwave treatments. J Agric Food Chem 2004 Dec 1;52(24):7318-23

4. Porter Y. Antioxidant properties of green broccoli and purple-sprouting broccoli under different cooking conditions. Bioscience Horizons (2012) 5: hzs004 doi: 10.1093/biohorizons/hzs004
5. Jaminet P. Do Microwaves destroy flavonoids? Retrieved from http://perfecthealthdiet.com/2010/12/do-microwaves-destroy-flavonoids/
6. Longo VD, Mattson MP. Fasting: molecular mechanisms and clinical applications. Cell Metab 2014 Feb 4;19(2):181-92
7. Horne BD, Muhlestein JB, May HT, Carlquist JF, Lappé DL, Bair TL, Anderson JL; Intermountain Heart Collaborative Study Group. Relation of routine, periodic fasting to risk of diabetes mellitus, and coronary artery disease in patients undergoing coronary angiography. Am J Cardiol 2012 Jun 1;109(11):1558-62
8. Environmental Working Group. 2014 Shopper's Guide to Pesticides in Produce. Retrieved from http://www.ewg.org/foodnews/summary.php
9. Campbell TC, Campbell TM. The China Study. Benbella Books, Texas. 2006

References for Chapter 18: Cancer concepts

1. Zu K, Mucci L, Rosner BA, Clinton SK, Loda M, Stampfer MJ, Giovannucci E. Dietary lycopene, angiogenesis, and prostate cancer: a prospective study in the prostate-specific antigen era. J Natl Cancer Inst 2014 Feb;106(2):djt430
2. LI WW. Can we eat to starve cancer? TED (Technology, Entertainment, Design) talk, 2010. Retrieved from www.ted.com/talks/william_li.html
3. LI WW, LI VW, Hutnik M, Chiou AS. Tumor angiogenesis as a target for dietary cancer prevention. J Oncol 2012;2012:879623
4. Stoner GD, Dombkowski AA, Reen RK, Cukovic D, Salagrama S, Wang LS, Lechner JF. Carcinogen-altered genes in rat esophagus positively modulated to normal levels of expression by both black raspberries and phenylethyl isothiocyanate. Cancer Res 2008 Aug 1;68(15):6460-7
5. Rakoff-Nahoum S. Why cancer and inflammation? Yale J Biol Med 2006 Dec;79(3-4):123-30
6. Coussens LM, Werb Z. Inflammation and cancer. Nature 2002 Dec 19-26;420(6917):860-7
7. Vendramini-Costa DB, Carvalho JE. Molecular link mechanisms between inflammation and cancer. Curr Pharm Des 2012;18(26):3831-52
8. Aggarwal BB, Shishodia S, Sandur SK, Pandey MK, Sethi G. Inflammation and cancer: how hot is the link? Biochem Pharmacol 2006 Nov 30;72(11):1605-21
9. Kundu JK, Surh YJ. Inflammation: gearing the journey to cancer. Mutat Res 2008 Jul-Aug;659(1-2):15-30
10. Ulrich CM, Bigler J, Potter JD. Non-steroidal anti-inflammatory drugs for cancer prevention: promise, perils and pharmacogenetics. Nat Rev Cancer 2006 Feb;6(2):130-40
11. Bellik Y, Boukraâ L, Alzahrani HA, Bakhotmah BA, Abdellah F, Hammoudi SM, Iguer-Ouada M. Molecular mechanism underlying

anti-inflammatory and anti-allergic activities of phytochemicals: an update. Molecules 2012 Dec 27;18(1):322-53

12. JI S. The dark side of wheat – new perspective on celiac disease and wheat intolerance. Retrieved from www.greenmedinfo.com/page/dark-side-wheat-new-perspectives-celiac-disease-wheat-intolerance-sayer-ji
13. Cloud J Why DNA Isn't Your Destiny. TIME Magazine, 6 January 2010. http://www.time.com/time/magazine/article/0,9171,1952313,00.html#ixzz1jbJjxmzy
14. Dolinoy DC, Weidman JR, Waterland RA, Jirtle RL. Maternal genistein alters coat color and protects Avy mouse offspring from obesity by modifying the fetal epigenome. Environ Health Perspect 2006 Apr;114(4):567-72
15. Meeran SM, Ahmed A, Tollefsbol TO. Epigenetic targets of bioactive dietary components for cancer prevention and therapy. Clin Epigenetics 2010 Dec 1;1(3-4):101-116
16. Huang J, Plass C, Gerhauser C. Cancer chemoprevention by targeting the epigenome. Curr Drug Targets 2011 Dec;12(13):1925-56
17. Anand P, Sundaram C, Jhurani S, Kunnumakkara AB, Aggarwal BB. Curcumin and cancer: an "old-age" disease with an "age-old" solution. Cancer Lett 2008 Aug 18;267(1):133-64
18. Surh Y-J, Chun K-S. Cancer chemopreventive effects of curcumin. Advances in experimental medicine and biology 2007;595:149-172
19. Campbell FC, Collett GP. Chemopreventive properties of curcumin. Future Oncol (2005)1(3):405–414
20. Aggarwal BB, Kumar A, Bharti AC. Anticancer potential of curcumin: preclinical and clinical studies. Anticancer Research 2003;23:363-398
21. Duvoix A, Blasius R, Delhalle S, Schnekenburger M, Morceau F, Henry E, Dicato M, Diederich M. Chemopreventive and therapeutic effects of curcumin. Cancer Letters 2005;223:181-190

References for Chapter 19: Research methods and major trials

1. Goldacre B. Bad Pharma: How drug companies mislead doctors and harm patients. 2012. HarperCollins, London
2. Boehm K, Borrelli F, Ernst E, Habacher G, Hung SK, Milazzo S, Horneber M. Green tea (Camellia sinensis) for the prevention of cancer (Review). In The Cochrane Collaboration. 2010, Issue 1. Published by JohnWiley & Sons, Ltd.
3. Gauch RR. It's Great! Oops, No It Isn't – Why clinical research can't guarantee the right medical answers. 2009. Springer
4. Smith-Warner SA, Spiegelman D, Yaun SS, Adami HO, Beeson WL, van den Brandt PA et al. Intake of fruits and vegetables and risk of breast cancer: a pooled analysis of cohort studies. JAMA 2001 Feb 14;285(6):769-76
5. Toniolo P, Van Kappel AL, Akhmedkhanov A, Ferrari P, Kato I, Shore RE, Riboli E. Serum carotenoids and breast cancer. Am J Epidemiol 2001 Jun 15;153(12):1142-7
6. Aune D, Chan DS, Vieira AR, Navarro Rosenblatt DA, Vieira R, Greenwood DC, Norat T. Dietary compared with blood concentrations of carotenoids

and breast cancer risk: a systematic review and meta-analysis of prospective studies. Am J Clin Nutr 2012 Aug;96(2):356-73

7. Rock CL, Flatt SW, Natarajan L, Thomson CA, Bardwell WA, Newman VA, Hollenbach KA, Jones L, Caan BJ, Pierce JP. Plasma carotenoids and recurrence-free survival in women with a history of breast cancer. J Clin Oncol 2005 Sep 20;23(27):6631-8
8. LI C, Ford ES, Zhao G, Balluz LS, Giles WH, Liu S. Serum α-carotene concentrations and risk of death among US Adults: the Third National Health and Nutrition Examination Survey Follow-up Study. Arch Intern Med. 2011 Mar 28;171(6):507-15
9. Eichholzer M, Stähelin HB, Gey KF, Lüdin E, Bernasconi F. Prediction of male cancer mortality by plasma levels of interacting vitamins: 17-year follow-up of the prospective Basel study. Int J Cancer 1996 Apr 10;66(2):145-50
10. Yuan JM, Ross RK, Gao YT, Qu YH, Chu XD, Yu MC. Prediagnostic levels of serum micronutrients in relation to risk of gastric cancer in Shanghai, China. Cancer Epidemiol Biomarkers Prev 2004 Nov;13(11 Pt 1):1772-80
11. Steinmetz KA, Kushi LH, Bostick RM, Folsom AR, Potter JD. Vegetables, fruit, and colon cancer in the Iowa Women's Health Study. Am J Epidemiol 1994 Jan 1;139(1):1-15
12. Chlebowski RT, Blackburn GL, Thomson CA, Nixon DW, Shapiro A, Hoy MK et al. Dietary fat reduction and breast cancer outcome: interim efficacy results from the Women's Intervention Nutrition Study. J Natl Cancer Inst 2006 Dec 20;98(24):1767-76
13. Prentice RL, Caan B, Chlebowski RT, Patterson R, Kuller LH, Ockene JK, Margolis KL et al. Low-fat dietary pattern and risk of invasive breast cancer: the Women's Health Initiative Randomized Controlled Dietary Modification Trial. JAMA 2006 Feb 8;295(6):629-42
14. Pierce JP, Natarajan L, Caan BJ, Parker BA, Greenberg ER, Flatt SW, Rock CL, Kealey S et al. Influence of a diet very high in vegetables, fruit, and fiber and low in fat on prognosis following treatment for breast cancer: the Women's Healthy Eating and Living (WHEL) randomized trial. JAMA 2007 Jul 18;298(3):289-98
15. Schulz M, Lahmann PH, Boeing H, Hoffmann K, Allen N, Key TJ, Bingham S, Wirfält E et al. Fruit and vegetable consumption and risk of epithelial ovarian cancer: the European Prospective Investigation into Cancer and Nutrition. Cancer Epidemiol Biomarkers Prev 2005 Nov;14(11 Pt 1):2531-5
16. van Gils CH, Peeters PH, Bueno-de-Mesquita HB, Boshuizen HC, Lahmann PH et al. Consumption of vegetables and fruits and risk of breast cancer. JAMA 2005 Jan 12;293(2):183-93
17. EPIC Project key findings. Retrieved from http://epic.iarc.fr/keyfindings.php
18. Benetou V, Trichopoulou A, Orfanos P, Naska A, Lagiou P, Boffetta P, Trichopoulos D; Greek EPIC cohort. Conformity to traditional Mediterranean diet and cancer incidence: the Greek EPIC cohort. Br J Cancer 2008 Jul 8;99(1):191-5

19. Wu AH, Yu MC, Tseng CC, Stanczyk FZ, Pike MC. Dietary patterns and breast cancer risk in Asian American women. Am J Clin Nutr 2009 Apr;89(4):1145-54

20. Boggs DA, Palmer JR, Wise LA, Spiegelman D, Stampfer MJ, Adams-Campbell LL, Rosenberg L. Fruit and vegetable intake in relation to risk of breast cancer in the Black Women's Health Study. Am J Epidemiol 2010 Dec 1;172(11):1268-79

21. Kirkegaard H, Johnsen NF, Christensen J, Frederiksen K, Overvad K, Tjønneland A. Association of adherence to lifestyle recommendations and risk of colorectal cancer: a prospective Danish cohort study. BMJ 2010 Oct 26;341:c5504

22. Willett WC, Hunter DJ, Stampfer MJ, Colditz G, Manson JE, Spiegelman D, Rosner B, Hennekens CH, Speizer FE. Dietary fat and fiber in relation to risk of breast cancer. An 8-year follow-up. JAMA 1992 Oct 21;268(15):2037-44

23. Baade PD, Meng X, Sinclair C, Youl P. Estimating the future burden of cancers preventable by better diet and physical activity in Australia. Med J Aust 2012 Mar 19;196(5):337-40

24. Cancer prevention and early detection (CPED) facts and figures 2011 (American Cancer Society) Retrieved from http://www.cancer.org/acs/groups/content/@epidemiologysurveilance/documents/document/acspc-029459.pdf

25. Parkin DM, Boyd L, Walker LC. The fraction of cancer attributable to lifestyle and environmental factors in the UK in 2010. Br J Cancer 2011 Dec 6;105 Suppl 2:S77-81

26. Cigarettes, diet, alcohol and obesity behind more than 100,000 cancers. Press release retrieved from www.cancerresearchuk.org/about-us/cancer-news/press-release/cigarettes-diet-alcohol-and-obesity-behind-more-than-100000-cancers

Printed in Great Britain
by Amazon

63172719R00132